Accreditation in the Health Sciences

MEDICAL LIBRARY ASSOCIATION BOOKS

The Medical Library Association (MLA) publishes state-of-the-art books that enhance healthcare, support professional development, improve library services, and promote research throughout the world.

MLA books are dynamic resources for librarians in hospitals, medical research practice, corporate libraries, and other settings. These invaluable publications provide medical librarians, healthcare professionals, and patients with accurate information that can improve outcomes and save lives.

MEDICAL LIBRARY ASSOCIATION BOOKS PANEL

The MLA Books Panel is responsible for (1) monitoring publishing trends within the industry; (2) exploring new concepts in publications by actively soliciting and proposing ideas for new publications; and (3) coordinating publishing efforts to achieve the best utilization of MLA resources. Each MLA book is directly administered from its inception by the MLA Books Panel, composed of MLA members with expertise spanning the breadth of health sciences librarianship.

ABOUT THE MEDICAL LIBRARY ASSOCIATION

The Medical Library Association (MLA) is a global, nonprofit educational organization with a membership of more than 400 institutions and 3,000 professionals in the health information field. Since 1898, MLA has fostered excellence in the professional practice and leadership of health sciences library and information professionals to enhance healthcare, education, and research throughout the world. MLA educates health information professionals, supports health information research, promotes access to the world's health sciences information, and works to ensure that the best health information is available to all.

RECENTLY PUBLISHED MLA BOOKS

3D Printing in Medical Libraries: A Crash Course in Supporting Innovation in Healthcare by Jennifer Herron

Diversity and Inclusion in Libraries: A Call to Action and Strategies for Success Edited by Shannon D. Jones and Beverly Murphy

Framing Health Care Instruction: An Information Literacy Handbook for the Health Sciences by Lauren M. Young and Elizabeth G. Hinton

The Clinical Medical Librarian's Handbook Edited by Judy C. Stribling

The Engaged Health Sciences Library Liaison Edited by Lindsay Alcock and Kelly Thormodson

A History of Medical Libraries and Medical Librarianship: From John Shaw Billings to the Digital Era by Michael R. Kronenfeld and Jennie Jacobs Kronenfeld

Planning and Promoting Events in Health Sciences Libraries: Success Stories and Best Practices Edited by Shalu Gillum and Natasha Williams

Great Library Events: From Planning to Promotion to Evaluation by Mary Grace Flaherty

Assessing Academic Library Performance: A Handbook by Holt Zaugg

Finding Your Seat at the Table: Roles for Librarians on Institutional Regulatory Boards and Committees Edited by Susan M. Harnett and Laureen P. Cantwell

Virtual Services in the Health Sciences Library: A Handbook Edited by Amanda R. Scull

Combating Online Health Misinformation: A Professional's Guide to Helping the Public Edited by Alla Keselman, Catherine Arnott Smith, and Amanda J. Wilson

Accreditation in the Health Sciences

A HANDBOOK

FOR LIBRARIANS

Edited by Darell Schmick

ROWMAN & LITTLEFIELD
Lanham • Boulder • New York • London

Disclaimer: Accreditation elements may be updated or changed at any time by accrediting agencies. As always, please refer to the accrediting agency for the latest requirements as they may have changed from the referenced elements in this book at time of publication.

Published by Rowman & Littlefield
An imprint of The Rowman & Littlefield Publishing Group, Inc.
4501 Forbes Boulevard, Suite 200, Lanham, Maryland 20706
www.rowman.com

86-90 Paul Street, London EC2A 4NE

British Library Cataloguing in Publication Information Available

Library of Congress Cataloging-in-Publication Data on File

ISBN 978-1-5381-6557-7 (cloth : alk. Paper)
ISBN 978-1-5381-6558-4 (electronic)

Contents

Acknowledgments

I would like to thank every author for their valuable contributions to this book. It was a pleasure to work with everyone who made this book richer by sharing their perspectives, advice, and wisdom. I thank Brandi Tuttle, and the Medical Library Association's Books Panel that she represents, for presenting us with the opportunity to make this book a reality; Erinn and Charles, for their patience and responsiveness when I had questions, and the rest of the team at Rowman & Littlefield; Roy Brown, who went above and beyond for his work and contributions—this book is undoubtedly a stronger book thanks to your efforts; my colleagues at Noorda College of Osteopathic Medicine, and in particular Deans Brown and Dougherty, for your enthusiastic support throughout this process. Finally, thank you so much to my mother, family, and friends for their unwavering support and for always rooting for me—your support means everything!

Introduction

Darell Schmick, Noorda College of Osteopathic Medicine

Accreditation is a word that can change the pace, tone, and timbre of a library's operations from top to bottom. The process is high stakes for the stakeholders that libraries serve, whether in a healthcare or academic setting. To best meet the needs of those groups going through accreditation, the library needs to understand the process and look for ways to be proactive and plan alongside those going through the process. If a library doesn't, the process can be one that can leave a library scrambling as it enters the accreditation process.

Entities that undergo accreditation may have to account for personnel, resources, and services, among many other dimensions. Libraries usually contain all three of the above criteria, so it would almost go without saying that an organization's library would be a vital part of the process.

The communications structures can vary significantly in health sciences organizations. Some libraries and their teams may benefit from excellent communication across the greater organization, and the process is relatively open. On the other end, the library is an afterthought, not-so-blissfully ignorant of the siloed structure and culture that prevent at least a meaningful interaction on the topic. This book was written to target all constituencies: big to small libraries, libraries that are brought close to their organizations on planning efforts and those that are still navigating through their institutional siloes. The lessons that follow will equip the readers with excellent ideas on how to move forward, no matter their library's situation.

Anyone who reads this book will be able to benefit from the knowledge that can be shared by the authors of each chapter—these chapters can stand alone as teaching lessons or be read collectively. The book is divided into three sections, which are clearly organized so that readers may quickly get to the information that may most directly pertain to what they are experiencing at the time. At the end of each section, there is a case study shared by one of their colleagues, a narrative designed to reinforce understandings presented in the prior chapters.

Part I discusses accreditation fundamentals. Why does an institution of learning and/or practice go through the trouble of accreditation, and where does the library fit, exactly? These chapters will provide a directed introduction, an overview of the accreditation process, and tried-and-true best practices for success—shared by fellow colleagues who have gone through the process before. In chapter 1, Dr. Norris writes about the history of accreditation in the United States and how it pertains to our constituencies. Chapter 2 will share accreditation preparation. How does one embark on preparing for such an event? This chapter will help you think about questions you will invariably need to answer as the process begins. The section will cap with how one library team found successes despite personnel changes at the greater institution and will share their results.

Part II will dive deeper into the actual accreditation process. At the time of writing, there are numerous colleges and universities ambitiously expanding their allied health programs. Are you at an institution that is just beginning a new program? Perhaps you were just hired at a school that is starting up a new medical school—surely a place where accreditation will be a focus. The section will begin by detailing lessons from experiencing a first-time accreditation process. Chapter 4's authors speak from experience and share their insights. Chapter 5 will detail an ongoing accreditation effort. Long-standing nursing magnet status at a top-tier institution? One of the oldest continuously operating medical schools in the country? This chapter will discuss the many opportunities in which a library can find renewed opportunities for partnership in these efforts. The next chapter shows how the library can illustrate the impact of meaningful continuous quality improvement (CQI) collaborations across campus. After all, our institutional improvements shouldn't just be a discussion exclusively among ourselves in the library! Chapter 7 interviews an experienced site inspector as they share insights from their perspective: what exactly are accrediting agencies looking for when they visit our institutions? This chapter will provide the practical advice that the library needs to be in the absolute best position to prepare for a site visit. This section also finishes with a relevant case study from the University of Mississippi to reinforce lessons from this section and share their best practices for accreditation success.

Part III summarizes the accreditation process. How can the library best wind down such an intensive, hands-on, and extensive effort? Chapter 9 discusses debriefing practices in detail, designed to equip the reader with practical information they can apply as their library wraps up its accreditation visit. Chapter 10 shares wisdom from a distinguished health sciences library director: how to deal with success as well as failure as institutions are born and grow. Sometimes an institution is successfully accredited or adequately accredited. Sometimes an institution does not meet standard. This chapter has been devoted to handling each of the contingencies and how to best prepare from where the library sits. Ensuring a proactive plan of action to follow an accreditation process—from initial reporting to site visit—is important to stay in the greater discussion, and that is covered in chapter 11. A final case study from an intrepid team at Georgetown weaving information-seeking skills to accreditation efforts caps this section to complete the book.

Having successfully completed several iterations of the accreditation process, at both established institutions and brand-new institutions and programs alike, I have long been perplexed as to why we don't have a professional manual designed to equip the reader with practical know-how and turn an involved, detail-rich event that all institutions go through and make it another strength from their library. It is my hope that this book capably prepares any library team to prepare well for any accreditation process.

Part One

Accreditation Fundamentals

1

Accrediting Bodies

HISTORY AND CONTEXT

Mitzi R. Norris, University of Mississippi Medical Center

A century ago, accreditation distinguished institutions with status and provided an important marketing advantage. Today, institutions of higher learning must attain the legal status of accreditation to satisfy the US Department of Education (USDOE) requirements and to qualify for federal financial aid. Additionally, the Higher Education Act uses accreditation as a means of quality assurance.

BEGINNING OF ACCREDITATION

For more than a century, academic accreditation has distinguished institutions of higher learning as representing a quality education. The first accrediting group, the New England Association of Schools and Colleges, was founded in 1885. Accrediting organizations were initially voluntary college associations. The expectations set by these associations resulted in standardization within colleges and universities across important categories such as library size, faculty size, and length of programs. The accredited status differentiated these institutions from other institutions of higher education that were not accredited, thus proving the superiority of accredited institutions.

Selden defined accreditation as "the process whereby an organization or agency recognizes a college or university or a program of study as having met certain pre-determined qualifications or standards."[1] Before the definition of accreditation became standardized, terms such as "registered," approved," "listed," and "eligible" were used.[2]

Harcleroad describes five time periods in the history of accreditation.[3] The first period, from 1787 to 1914, provided structure, much of which continues today. In 1787 the first recognition was from the New York Regents that was required by law to visit and review each college in the state every year. The institutions were identified as "registered." Other states later adopted a similar structure. In 1847 the American Medical Association represented programmatic accreditation, and these associations began. In 1912 one of the regional accreditors established the twelve specific criteria for accreditation. Additionally, in 1914 the Association of American Universities (AAU) developed and published a list grouping institutions by educational quality.

During the second period, from 1914 to 1935, more organizations established accreditation criteria, and national associations began in 1926. The third period, from 1935 to 1948, saw growth in specialized accreditation organizations such as an organization for libraries (1924) and the Liaison Committee on Medical Education. States also established standards and state accreditation of institutions. One of the objectives of the state involvement in accreditation was to thwart diploma mills. The regional accreditors realigned the basics of accreditation to recognize the individual institution's objectives rather than a single set of criteria. The change positioned these organizations to adapt to diverse institutions.

In the fourth period, from 1948 to 1975, the AAU discontinued the ranking on the quality of institutions, and the number of specialized accrediting organizations increased rapidly. The major element of the time period was the development of the federal role in accreditation. The influence was established to oversee federal funding of institutions and funding to students. Additionally, in 1952 the GI Bill for Korean War veterans was reauthorized.[3,4] The 1944 Servicemen's Readjustment Act (GI Bill)[4,5] provided financial aid directly to veterans to pay for training and education. However, this led to shoddy programs. As a result, the 1952 bill required institutions receiving funds from the GI Bill be recognized as accredited by organizations included in the USDOE list of accrediting and state organizations.[5,6]

The final period listed in Harcleroad's history[7] of accreditation was from 1975 to 1980. During this period, organizations developed to oversee accreditors and worked to minimize federal efforts to turn voluntary membership associations into policing organizations. The period ushered in the federal use of accreditation to protect education consumers and to incorporate social equity goals.

PURPOSE OF ACCREDITATION

Although early reasons for accreditation may have appeared superficial, the prevailing purpose of accreditation today is to validate quality programs and to provide accountability to students, parents, financial funders, and potential employers.

To provide a quality education for students, institutions must be vigilant in maintaining high standards for academic programs. Accreditation validates that goal. Accreditation demonstrates how programs measure against commonly accepted standards.

Such standardization provided the means for students to transfer from one institution to another. The process recognized a consistent measure of education, the credit hour. Accreditation organizations were established to determine admission of high school graduates by diploma rather than examination and to establish and maintain academic standards.[8] The process also describes resources to help students succeed. The number of faculty and qualification of faculty were examined during the accreditation process. Additionally, resources such as the adequacy of the library were evaluated. Some accreditors noted the number of books available for faculty and students. These measures served to validate program quality at accredited institutions.

Accreditation also provides transparency to the benefactors and funders of higher education. In the federally funded study of accreditation by Orlans,[9] the USDOE defined accreditation as "the voluntary process whereby and agency or association grants public recognition to a school, institute, college, university, or specialized program of study that meets certain established qualification and educational standards . . . as determined through initial and periodic evaluations."

Accreditation is a legal status.[10] For federal purposes, the status allows students at accredited postsecondary institutions to use federal funds to pay for their education. USDOE requires students who receive federal loans, work-study, and Pell grants to attend accredited institutions. The most recent numbers from the National Advisory Committee on Institutional Quality and Integrity (NACIQI)[11] indicate about 48 percent of 15.6 million undergraduate students received federal loans. Students and/or parents who pay tuition or repay loans can use the transparency of accreditation to determine the value of the education.

Student achievement data are a part of the accreditation process. Student achievement statistics are consistently defined metrics that students and other stakeholders can use to judge the appropriateness of the cost of education. For professions that require licensure, tracking a program's success at equipping students based on a standard test is a good benchmark of a program's quality.[12] For instance, students and parents would want to review a program's nursing licensure pass rate before committing time and funds to the program.

Employers, as consumers of graduates of educational programs, are uniquely interested in the track record of an institution. Programs that consistently graduate students who have the skills employers need provide a reasonable predictive algorithm for success of other graduates. Thus, these programs establish a pipeline for companies to hire competent workers and, conversely, for students to have a ready option for employment post-graduation.[13]

Institutional autonomy is recognized as an important element for institutions to control academic quality. Consequently, accreditation standards protect institutions from external and internal pressures. Academic freedom is also part of the expectation to promote a quality education for students.[14]

At its best, accreditation is a continuous quality improvement process. Institutions measure themselves against accreditation standards during the self-study process. During this time, the prudent institution uses the process to make adjustments and improvements. As gaps in process, procedures, services, or activities are identified, institutions can implement changes to rectify the discrepancy. The process improves academic programs and strengthens the academic mission of the institution. During a recent self-study accreditation process, an institution tracked actions that changed or improved processes. Forty-one improvements were made. The scrutiny of the self-study clarifies areas to improve. The changes improve the institution and the academic programs; therefore, accreditation benchmarks the achievement of educational standards. The scrutiny of accreditation is important for credibility and accountability to students and other stakeholders.

PROCESS OF ACCREDITATION

The Council of Higher Education Accreditation (CHEA)[15] defines accreditation in higher education as "a collegial process based on self and peer assessment for public accountability and improvement of academic quality."

Accreditation is comprised primarily of five areas:[16] self-study, peer review, site visit, action/judgment, and monitoring/oversight.

SELF-STUDY

Accreditation evaluates an institution based on an established set of criteria. The institution or program participates in a self-study. Faculty, staff, and administrators contribute to the study in their area of expertise. The information from the self-assessment provides the institution's or program's narrative about how the threshold is met. The accreditation process is focused on the institution's or program's mission, thus recognizing the uniqueness of institutions and programs.[17]

Some of the standards within institutional accreditation are directed by requirements of the USDOE. These are basic questions about facilities, faculty, resources, and curriculum. Accreditation is a nongovernment self-regulation process that occurs on a cycle—usually five to ten years.

PEER REVIEW/SITE VISIT

The accreditation process[18] for an institution or program is conducted by a team of peers. These individuals review the institution's or program's self-study and then visit the location to validate information and review the physical resources. Institutional accreditation is comprehensive and includes finance, governance, student services, faculty, resources, and student learning and achievement. Programmatic accreditation includes standards that are more targeted to the specific discipline but also look at overarching context, such as mission.

ACTION/JUDGMENT

After reviewing the self-study and completing a site visit, a team of peers writes a report of the findings based on a set of expectations for quality and integrity that guide the process. The report is a legal document attesting to the condition of the institution and a judgment about how the institution meets the thresholds required by the accrediting body.

MONITORING/OVERSIGHT

Accreditation is a continuous process. After initial accreditation, institutions and programs must undergo the reaccreditation process on a regular basis. Between review cycles, institutions are required to provide information about significant changes such as a change in governance. Programmatic accreditors also require updates about significant events, and some require annual updates.[19]

OVERSIGHT OF THE ACCREDITATION PROCESS

The USDOE and the Council for Higher Education Accreditation (CHEA) are the primary accreditation agencies to determine whether institutions of higher education are accredited.[20] USDOE and CHEA approve accreditation associations. They do not accredit institutions or programs. The USDOE uses an institution's accreditation status to qualify schools to receive federal financial aid.

The USDOE and the CHEA review accreditation agencies to determine if those agencies meet the quality standards of their respective organizations. The primary purpose of USDOE recognition of accrediting agencies is to assure the use of federal student aid funds on quality programs. The primary purpose of CHEA recognition of accrediting agencies is to assure and strengthen academic quality while documenting ongoing improvement in academic programs. The USDOE process is governed by federal law and regulations. CHEA, a private organization, is governed by a board of directors.[21]

NACIQI monitors the academic quality of institutions and programs for federal purposes. NACIQI advises the US secretary of education on accreditation and recommends recognition of accrediting organizations to USDOE. Members are appointed by the secretary of education and are not a part of the governmental process. The USDOE must approve associations before the institutions accredited by the organizations can be eligible to participate in federal programs such as student financial assistance.[22]

Accrediting organizations must themselves be reviewed periodically.[23] The review process is to confirm that the organizations have processes and outcomes in place to protect students and the public. USDOE or CHEA are the primary organizations to provide this oversight. Accrediting associations that meet the standards are deemed "recognized."

The basic structure of accreditation[24] is described as "triad." The three elements are state governments, voluntary accreditation associations, and the federal government. State governments incorporate the institutions that provide education and licensed individuals in certain occupations and professions. Additionally, some states have groups with legal authority to accredit institutions and programs.

Voluntary accreditation associations are organizations that accredit institutions or programs. Institutional organizations have national or regional oversight.[25]

The federal part of accreditation is derived from the taxing and spending authorization. The federal government provides funds to institutions that are "eligible" to receive funding and to students who attend "eligible" institutions. Thus, the federal USDOE and private CHEA recognize accreditors who meet established thresholds. These organizations in turn accredit programs or institutions.

TYPES OF ACCREDITING ORGANIZATIONS

There are four types of US accrediting organizations:[26] regional, national faith-related, national career-related, and programmatic.

REGIONAL ACCREDITORS

The first type, the regional accreditors, have US geographical boundaries. These organizations accredit public, private, two- and four-year institutions. The regional institutional portfolio consists mainly of nonprofit and degree-granting institutions. Institutional accreditation is comprehensive.[27]

The six regional accreditors were primarily founded in the late 1800s as voluntary organizations. Over time, these accreditors moved to standardized metrics such as library size, number of faculty, length of programs of study, and transferability of credits. These improvements were marketing tools to distinguish accredited institutions from those not meeting the standards.[28]

The initial regional organizations were recently reclassified. The term "regional" can be omitted; these organizations are no longer geographically bound. In 2019 the USDOE entered into negotiated rule making about the types of accreditations.[29] The result was the decision that regional accreditors could be free to accredit anywhere in the United States, thus changing the footprint. USDOE stated the goal was to open the institutional accreditation system to competition. The decision to change to include other geographic areas is the decision of the regional accreditor. One by one, each regional organization has opened the borders to expand its geographic imprint.

Judith Eaton, past president of CHEA, discussed the positives and negatives about regional accreditors' new freedom to become national. Four reasons were identified to remain regional.[30] First is the unique composition of the region's institutional mix. For example, almost two-thirds of New England institutions are private, while more than half of the institutions in the middle of the country are public.

The second point references the cultures of the regions. While standards are similar, the values and focus of institutions have different emphasis. The third reason is practical and financial. The geographic differences can add workload and cost. Institutions deciding to change to another accreditor will incur additional expenses. The fourth reason identifies the possibility of institutions shopping around for an easier accreditor, thus lowering the expectations of this self-regulated process.

Dr. Eaton also identifies four reasons why accreditors' changing from regional is positive. The first is that regional accreditors already operate outside the geographic lines by accrediting institutions with online learning and branch or off-site campuses. Some of the regionals also accredit international institutions.

The second reason is increased growth opportunities. Without geographically limits, organizations would strengthen the importance and impact of regional accreditation. Third, the change would broaden regional organizations' creative and innovation possibilities. The fourth reason is that competition could strengthen accreditation.

NATIONAL ACCREDITORS

The second and third types of accrediting organizations can be grouped as national accreditors. This group includes both faith-related accreditors and career-related accreditors. The faith-related are religious institutions that are generally nonprofit and degree granting. The career-related accreditors, on the other hand, are primarily for-profit, single-purpose institutions that can either be degree granting or non–degree granting.

The faith-related organizations began out of a need for recognition and followed a course much like the regional and programmatic accreditors. Because these organizations are usually affiliated with a religious organization, accreditation can revolve around the question of independence from the parent denomination.

The national career-related accrediting organizations developed as a need to assert that the organization contributed to the public good. These accredit programs that provide a credential in a specialized field. The accreditation usually relates to employment in a specialized career. Because of the proprietary nature of these institutions, these accreditors have more frequently been the subject of investigations of fraud.[31]

PROGRAMMATIC ACCREDITORS

The fourth type of accreditor is programmatic. In addition to campus-wide accreditation, colleges and universities use programmatic accreditation to validate the institution's adherence to commonly accepted standards within specialized disciplines.

Programmatic accreditors accredit discipline-specific programs such as law or medicine. These accreditors developed in an unfolding fashion, much like the regional accreditors. These emerged from professional societies, and many of them were health related.

Vibert notes that programmatic accreditors are reliant on community and employers as an element of the accreditation process.[32] These individuals hold programs to industry standards and help programs benchmark against working best practices. Additionally, programmatic accreditors focus on professional competencies students are expected to obtain within the program of study. Student learning outcomes measure these essential elements.

A critical piece of medical accreditation history is found in the Flexner Report.[33] In November 1908, the trustees of the Carnegie Foundation authorized a study of the medicine and law schools in the United States. Abraham Flexner was identified to examine medical education. The result transformed medical education that until that point had admitted students with few or no standards for a few months of study with an apprenticeship before being awarded a doctor of medicine degree.

Findings of the study concluded that for the past twenty-five years there had been an overproduction of uneducated and ill-trained medical practitioners. Public welfare was not considered. Many of the existing medical schools were commercial entities sustained by advertising. The curriculum of the schools was primarily didactic, with inadequate laboratories because of the cost. The report stated that a hospital under complete educational control was necessary for medical training, as were laboratories for chemistry and pathology.

The report stated, "It is clear that so long as a man is to practice medicine, the public is equally concerned in his right preparation for that profession." Within ten years of the report's release, the number of medical schools was reduced by almost half (162 to 85), and almost all of the remaining schools were associated with a university. Selden described the progress made by medical education during this time, which included the development of standards and expectation.[34] Selden concluded that accreditation improved medical education.

THE LIBRARY'S ROLE IN ACCREDITATION

Institutional library resources are one of the pillars of academic accreditation. The library's role is to provide adequate resources and services to students and faculty. A hallmark of all types of academic accreditation is an examination of the resources and services of libraries. The Higher Education Act of 1965 was a law to strengthen educational resources such as libraries at colleges and universities and to provide financial assistance for students.[35]

Institutional accreditors include standards that examine library holdings and space. Accreditors also examine the role and availability of libraries to serve faculty and students. Libraries are required to have adequate resources related to specific programs of study. These are evaluated with both institutional and programmatic accreditation.

In her book *Promises Kept,* Janis Quinn describes the importance of library holdings to accreditation.[36] The University of Mississippi was found noncompliant based on the lack of volumes in the library. Peter Whitman Rowland, MD, professor of pharmacology, assumed the responsibility of populating the library. To accomplish this, he rode in his pickup truck around the state, asking recent graduates to contribute their textbook. He was successful, and the institution was reaccredited. Today, library accreditation standards evaluate the adequacy of appropriate references to serve academic programs.

SUMMARY

Accreditation was established to identify institutions that met specified standards. Dr. Judith Eaton, the leading voice of accreditation, was asked during an interview about the purpose of accreditation. Her comments summarize the role of accreditation. Dr. Eaton stated, "To me, accreditation is a combination of quality assurance that is threshold quality, accountability for quality, and quality improvement. I know that the origins of accreditation put a primary focus on quality improvement—making things better. I think in today's world and going forward, accountability for quality is at least as important."

The process of accreditation provides accountability to students and the public about the quality of educational programs. The process provides a basis for the government to provide federal funds to students. Libraries continue to play an important role in the overall institutional accreditation. Libraries fulfill a unique role in programmatic accreditation in the health sciences.

NOTES

1. William K. Selden, *Accreditation: A Struggle for Standards in Higher Education.* (New York: Harper & Brothers, 1960).
2. Fred F. Harcleroad, "Accreditation: History, Process, and Problems," AAHE-ERIC/ Higher Education Research Report No. 6, 1980.
3. Harcleroad, "Accreditation."
4. Council for Higher Education Accreditation (CHEA), "The Fundamentals of Accreditation," September 2002.
5. Program on Education Policy and Governance, Harvard Kennedy School, "College Accreditation, Explained," *Education Next* (June 13, 2018): 1–10.
6. Peter T. Ewell, *U.S. Accreditation and the Future of Quality Assurance* (Washington, DC: Council on Higher Education Institute for Research and Study of Accreditation and Quality Assurance, 2008), 40.

7. Harcleroad, "Accreditation."
8. Selden, *Accreditation*, 42.
9. Harold Orlans, "The End of a Monopoly?" *Change* 12, no. 2 (February-March 1980): 32–37.
10. Program on Education Policy and Governance, "College Accreditation" 1–10.
11. National Advisory Committee on Institutional Quality and Integrity (NACIQ), "Dashboard," Meeting July 27–29, 2021, https://sites.ed.gov/naciqi/.
12. CHEA, "What is Accreditation?" February 1998.
13. Judith S. Eaton, "Accreditation in the United States," *New Directions for Higher Education* 145 (Spring 2009): 79–86.
14. Judith S. Eaton, "An Overview of U.S. Accreditation," Council for Higher Education Accreditation, revised November 2015.
15. CHEA, "What Is Accreditation?"
16. CHEA, "Fundamentals."
17. CHEA, "What Is Accreditation?"
18. CHEA, "What Is Accreditation?"
19. CHEA, "Fundamentals."
20. Eaton, "Accreditation," 79–86.
21. CHEA, "Fundamentals."
22. Ewell, *U.S. Accreditation*, 80–104.
23. Council for Higher Education Accreditation, "The Value of Accreditation," June 2010.
24. Harcleroad, "Accreditation."
25. Harcleroad,"Accreditation."
26. Eaton, "Overview."
27. CHEA, "What is Accreditation?"
28. Program on Education Policy and Governance, "College Accreditation," 1–10.
29. Judith S. Eaton, "Will Regional Accreditation Go National?" *Inside Higher Education*, March 17, 2020, https://www.insidehighered.com/views/2020/03/17/pros-and-cons-having-regional-accreditors-go-national-opinion.
30. Eaton, "Will Regional Accreditation Go National?"
31. Ewell, *U.S. Accreditation*, 80–104.
32. Joseph Vibert, "The Evolving Contest of Quality Assurance," in *Accreditation on the Edge*, ed. Susan D. Phillips and Devin Kinser (Baltimore: Johns Hopkins University Press, 2018), 44–63.
33. Abraham Flexner, "Medical Education in the United States and Canada," Bulletin 4 (New York: Carnegie Foundation, 1910).
34. Selden, *Accreditation*, 57–58.
35. J. McCants, "Do You Know TRIO?" *National TRIO Clearinghouse—Council for Opportunity in Education* 2 (February 2003).
36. Janis Quinn, *Promises Kept* (Jackson: University Press of Mississippi, 2005).

BIBLIOGRAPHY

Council for Higher Education Accreditation. "What Is Accreditation?" February 1998.

———. "The Fundamentals of Accreditation." September 2002.

———. "The Value of Accreditation." June 2010.

Eaton, Judith S. "Accreditation in the United States." *New Directions for Higher Education* 145 (Spring 2009): 79–86.

———. "An Overview of U.S. Accreditation," Council for Higher Education Accreditation, revised November 2015.

———. "Will Regional Accreditation Go National?" *Inside Higher Education* (March 17, 2020). https://www.insidehighered.com/views/2020/03/17/pros-and-cons-having-regional-accreditors-go-national-opinion.

Ewell, Peter T. *U.S. Accreditation and the Future of Quality Assurance*. Washington, DC: Council on Higher Education Institute for Research and Study of Accreditation and Quality Assurance, 2008.

Flexner, Abraham. "Medical Education in the United States and Canada." Bulletin 4. New York: Carnegie Foundation, 1910.

Harcleroad, Fred F. "Accreditation: History, Process, and Problems." AAHE-ERIC/Higher Education Research Report No. 6, 1980.

McCants, J. "Do You Know TRIO?" *National TRIO Clearinghouse—Council for Opportunity in Education* 2 (February 2003).

National Advisory Committee on Institutional Quality and Integrity (NACIQI). "Dashboard." Meeting July 27–29, 2021. https://sites.ed.gov/naciqi/.

Orlans, Harold. "The End of a Monopoly?" *Change* 12, no. 2 (February–March 1980): 32–37.

Program on Education Policy and Governance, Harvard Kennedy School. "College Accreditation, Explained." *Education Next* (June 13, 2018).

Quinn, Janis. *Promises Kept*. Jackson: University Press of Mississippi, 2005.

Selden, William K. *Accreditation: A Struggle for Standards in Higher Education*. New York: Harper & Brothers, 1960.

Vibert, Joseph. "The Evolving Contest of Quality Assurance." In *Accreditation on the Edge*, edited by Susan D. Phillips and Devin Kinser, 44–63. Baltimore: Johns Hopkins University Press, 2018.

2

Library Preparation for Accreditation

Roy Brown, Virginia Commonwealth University

Healthcare today is a complex environment with an ever-growing number of demands placed upon those tasked with providing care to those who need it most. The demands on the system arise from the communities served, patients, patients' families, insurance companies/payers, and government entities at both the state and federal levels. These demands are often translated to organizations in the form of accreditation standards that organizations must adhere to in order to continue operating or be viewed as trusted organizations. Accreditation standards/criteria exist at the national, state, and regional levels. In the clinical setting, patient safety is the primary focus. Clinical accreditation aims to decrease variation in practice, eliminate unnecessary care or tests, and ensure cost-effective care.[1] In the academic arena, the purpose is to ensure that educational programs prepare students for patient care upon graduation. These standards affect the libraries supporting the healthcare organizations and those schools that educate future healthcare practitioners. The demands that libraries face related to accreditation stem from stakeholders' expectations going through accreditation and from accreditation standards specifically related to libraries.

ACCREDITATION STANDARDS

There are many different accrediting organizations with different focuses and requirements. Depending on the set of standards in question, the role of libraries may or may not be explicitly stated. Even if a standard mentions the library, it may be generally written. For example, the standards may note that library resources and services should be available. As to the quality of those resources or services, the expectations may be just as general. It could be a statement that just states that resources and services need to be adequate to meet the needs of clinicians, students, faculty, or the educational program.[2] This lack of specificity or omission is not detrimental to a library being involved in the accreditation process. Instead, it should be viewed as an opportunity by a library. The library, together with stakeholders, can identify opportunities for the library to be involved in meeting accreditation standards. This will enable a library to show a return on investment and further demonstrate its value to a particular program, discipline, or organization. The value of the library could be derived from the collection, resources, and services the library provides. The services provided could include interlibrary loan services, participating in course-integrated instruction,[3,4] clinical rounds,[5,6,7,8] participating in an organization's evidence-based practice and quality improvement processes,[9,10,11,12,13] or creating an institutional repository to capture various projects.[14]

Accreditation standards tend to fall into two categories: (1) healthcare facility accreditation (hospitals, ambulatory care clinics, etc.) and (2) academic-oriented accreditation. Understanding which accreditation standards may affect a particular library is critical. Healthcare facility accreditation focuses on clinical care and patient safety. Academic-oriented accreditation focuses on the educational preparation of healthcare practitioners in a specific discipline. These accreditation standards aim to ensure that those who graduate are prepared to care for patients.

Accreditation is a voluntary process that an organization decides to participate in to demonstrate the quality of its practices and procedures. While accreditation is voluntary, outside entities like federal and state governments, private insurance companies, and other regulating bodies may have requirements that make it difficult to operate without accreditation. Furthermore, many professional organizations in the healthcare disciplines like the American Medical Association (AMA), the American Dental Association (ADA), and the American Nurses Association (ANA) require it for graduates of educational programs to practice.

Accredited healthcare facilities benefit from the designation, as accreditation makes them eligible for government funding through programs like Medicare and Medicaid. It may also allow the organization to participate in other government programs and qualify for other funding types. It is also a designation that private insurance companies want from those organizations that wish to be reimbursed for their patient care services.

Accreditation is a state requirement in many states for the schools that prepare future healthcare practitioners. Aside from the state requirement, students receive federal financial aid and sit for their licensure exam upon graduation. If a student attends an accredited institution, they are eligible to receive federal financial aid and sit for their licensure exam upon graduation.

HEALTHCARE FACILITY ACCREDITATION

To best demonstrate how the library impacts clinical care in a healthcare facility, libraries and librarians must understand the accreditation process and the standards. An excellent initial step in understanding the accreditation process is to become familiar with the accreditation standards that need to be met. Finding the library's place in these standards is complicated when the stakeholder is a healthcare facility; the library is tasked with serving many healthcare professionals from different disciplines, each with different needs. In addition, accreditation is made more complex when there are no physical or virtual library accreditation requirements established by those who accredit healthcare facilities.[15] Librarians in these settings must understand that the focus is on government compliance and accreditation standards. This focus is driven by the Centers for Medicare and Medicaid Services (CMS), which provide healthcare coverage to Americans by overseeing Medicare, Medicaid, the Children's Health Insurance Program, and the Health Insurance Marketplace.[16] Along with private insurance, it is also one of the big payers in the system, which provides CMS with a great deal of influence. According to the organization's strategic plan, CMS aims to accomplish six things: advance equity, expand access, engage partners, drive innovation, protect programs, and foster excellence.[17] Understanding these standards established by CMS can help libraries get a sense of where they can provide value to the organization.

To achieve its goals, CMS uses the eligibility to receive funding through Medicare and other funding to meet specific requirements. These requirements or standards are administered at the state level through Quality Improvement Organizations (QIOs). QIOs are composed of a group of health quality experts, clinicians, and consumers organized to improve the quality of care as mandated by CMS. Two types of QIOs focus on different aspects of healthcare. The Beneficiary and Family Centered Care (BFCC) QIOs oversee standards related to patients by addressing complaints and providing quality of care reviews. The Quality Innovation Network (QIN) QIOs aim to improve healthcare by utilizing data to improve patient safety, make communities healthier, coordinate post-hospital care, and improve clinical quality.[18]

CMS requires facilities receiving funds to undergo a review by a state survey agency or CMS-approved organization. Some healthcare facilities utilize state survey agencies to meet CMS requirements. These agencies carry out annual inspections to ensure healthcare facilities have policies and staff to provide quality care. However, this route is not one that most hospitals or healthcare organizations take to ensure alignment with CMS requirements. Those who choose this route tend to be smaller and in rural settings that lack an intensive care unit and teaching focus.[19]

The state survey agency route is not the path for most healthcare facilities. Healthcare facilities instead contract with private organizations to achieve accreditation. Approximately 75 percent of healthcare facilities take this route to accreditation. These organizations use trained peer reviewers to examine the quality of the organizational activities over a designated period. As a result, libraries are more likely to be a part of an organization that participates in an accreditation process administered by a private organization like the Joint Commission. The accreditation standards of these private organizations are aimed at meeting CMS requirements (see table 2.1).[20,21]

CMS is not the only driver of accreditation activities in a healthcare facility. Other accrediting bodies have standards that place additional requirements on an organization. One group of accrediting bodies with additional requirements focuses on medical education and practice. These organizations are the Liaison Committee on Medical Education (LCME), the Accreditation Council for Continuing Medical Education (ACCME), and the Accreditation Council for Graduate Medical Education (ACGME). Libraries play a role in meeting these standards and are often active through instructional services and the library collection.[22,23,24]

The Commission on Accreditation of Rehabilitation Facilities (CARF) and the ANCC Magnet Recognition Program are other accrediting bodies that set additional demands on healthcare facilities. These two bodies have standards that focus on the quality and safety of patient care. CARF is an organization that focuses on providing accreditation of those services across the continuum of care that serves children to seniors. CARF accredits many types of living and care options. These include addiction and substance abuse treatment, rehabilitation after an injury or disease, employment for persons with a disability, child welfare services, home and community services, and retirement living.[25] While not all of these settings are ones that libraries may have a role in as part of a healthcare facility, some healthcare organizations do provide these services. Having some knowledge of these accreditation standards is another way for libraries to meet the needs of stakeholders and further demonstrate value.

Table 2.1. CMS-Approved Accrediting Organizations

Accrediting Organization	*Website*
The Joint Commission (TJC)	https://www.jointcommission.org/
DNV GL Healthcare (DNV)	https://www.dnv.us/assurance/healthcare
Accreditation Commission for Health Care (ACHC)	https://www.achc.org/
Center for Improvement in Healthcare Quality (CIHQ)	https://www.cihq.org/

The ANCC Magnet Recognition Program is focused on nursing practice. This program is an accreditation many hospitals pursue; it is viewed as a method to empower nurses, improve patient care, and improve nurse retention. The empowerment of nurses in the program is driven by the program's mission to bring about excellence through leadership, scientific discovery, and the dissemination and implementation of new knowledge.[26] This focus on discovering and using evidence makes evidence-based practice (EBP) a crucial part of nursing practice in these organizations. EBP is where libraries can demonstrate their value to the organization through the collection and services that address this activity.

This is especially true because a part of the program is the Vizient/AACN Nurse Residency Program, a transition to practice program for new graduate nurses. This program is focused on acclimating them to the clinical practice environment. In addition, the program focuses on leadership, patient outcomes, and professional development. These three things are brought together to help nurses impact patient care through the expectation that each nurse resident is expected to participate in an EBP project to further their knowledge and address an issue in the clinical setting.[27]

ACADEMIC ACCREDITATION

Libraries involved in the accreditation process regarding future healthcare professionals' academic and clinical preparation may find it a bit easier to identify where the library can support accreditation. This is mainly because the standards will at least address the library collection. That is not to say that library services around course-integrated instruction and other contributions to a particular school's curriculum are not valued. It is just that these activities are not usually explicitly mentioned. However, the mention of the library in the accreditation standards provides libraries an opportunity to show the value recognized by not only the school served but also those who make accreditation site visits. Depending on the school(s) served by a particular library, several sets of standards may need to be reviewed. This number is driven by the fact that each discipline has its own accreditation standards that are aimed at best preparing future practitioners. Some of the most common accrediting organizations are listed in table 2.2 by discipline.

Table 2.2. Academic/Discipline-Specific Accrediting Agencies*

Discipline	*Accrediting Organization*	*Website*
Medicine	Liaison Committee on Medical Education (LCME)	https://www.aamc.org/services/first-for-financial-aid-officers/lcme-accreditation
	Accreditation Council for Continuing Medical Education (ACCME)	https://www.accme.org/
	Accreditation Council for Graduate Medical Education (ACGME)	https://www.acgme.org/
Osteopathic Medicine	Commission on Osteopathic College Accreditation	https://osteopathic.org/accreditation/
Physician Assistants	The Accreditation Review Commission on Education for the Physician Assistant (ARC-PA)	http://www.arc-pa.org/
Nursing	Accreditation Commission for Education in Nursing	https://www.acenursing.org/
	Commission on Collegiate Nursing Education (CCNE)	https://www.aacnnursing.org/CCNE
Pharmacy	Accreditation Council for Pharmacy Education (ACPE)	https://www.acpe-accredit.org/
Dentistry	Commission on Dental Accreditation (CODA)	https://www.acpe-accredit.org/
Public Health	Council of Education for Public Health	https://ceph.org/
Nursing Anesthesia	Council on Accreditation of Nurse Anesthesia Educational Programs (COA)	https://www.coacrna.org/

Discipline	*Accrediting Organization*	*Website*
Occupational Therapy	Accreditation Council for Occupational Therapy Education	https://acoteonline.org/
Physical Therapy	Commission on Accreditation in Physical Therapy Education (CAPTE)	https://www.capteonline.org/
Radiation Science	Joint Review Committee on Education in Radiologic Technology	https://www.jrcert.org/
Health Administration	Commission on Accreditation of Healthcare Management Education	https://www.cahme.org/
Counseling	Association for Counselor Education and Supervision (ACES)	https://www.cacrep.org/
Medical Laboratory Sciences	National Accrediting Agency for Clinical Laboratory Sciences (NAACLS)	https://www.naacls.org/about.aspx
Gerontology	Accreditation for Gerontology Education Council (AGEC)	http://www.geroaccred.org/

**This list is not intended to be exhaustive but an example of accrediting agencies for various health sciences disciplines.*

THE ACCREDITATION PROCESS: TAKING IT STEP BY STEP

The accreditation process is a multistep process where a school or healthcare facility's procedures, structures, processes, and policies are reviewed by an external body. Meeting these standards communicates to both internal and external stakeholders that the organization is operating at a high level with a continual focus on improving the quality of patient care or the education received by students.

An organization goes through a full accreditation cycle that can range from two to ten years. The accreditation process typically entails submitting data and reports that address specific accreditation standards and culminating in a site visit by the external reviewers. Some accrediting organizations only visit at the end of the accreditation cycle, while others may make site visits throughout the process. If a visit must be made before the culminating visit, it will be announced.

The only exception to this may be healthcare facilities. Healthcare facilities are also subject to unannounced visits or visits conducted with short notice. An example is the Joint Commission, which subjects healthcare facilities going through accreditation to unannounced and announced visits. In other cases, these visits may come on short notice for a setting where an unannounced visit is not feasible. In this case, the facility may get a week's notice that a visit is coming.[28] These visits would not typically involve the library but are done to evaluate clinical practice.

Accreditation can be overwhelming and cannot be done well without a plan. Knowing the timeline of an accreditation cycle will allow a library to develop a plan to provide the needed information. It also allows the library to determine if the library collection, resources, and services align with the standards. Many organizations approach this process like any other big project: by adopting sound project management processes and breaking the accreditation cycle down into small steps or tasks. An example would be a four-year accreditation cycle that breaks down the process by year. Libraries should mirror this approach to ensure that standards can be met and that the library can devote adequate and timely resources to ensure success.

YEAR 1: ESTABLISHING THE FOUNDATION FOR SUCCESS

The first year of the process can set the organization and library up for success if there is a thoughtful and strategic plan. The accreditation cycle starts with the organization identifying which accrediting body is appropriate and reviewing the standards. Next, a library must review these standards. Some accreditation standards are easy to access as they are posted on the accrediting body's website, while others must be purchased. Certain standards come with a cost to access. This is a cost the library may not want to take on; it can be expensive. This cost makes it essential that a library be engaged with the stakeholders going through the accreditation process. These stakeholders will have a copy of the standards and may provide them to the library or at least provide the opportunity to review them. During this early review of the standards, the library must identify and engage those stakeholders to determine their expectations regarding the library and the accreditation process. Understanding the library collection, resources, and services expectations are essential. Understanding these expectations is significant because the library may or may not be mentioned in the accreditation standards. As mentioned before, the omission of the library from accreditation standards can serve as an opportunity. During discussions with stakeholders, the library may also be able to point out where the library can further support the accreditation process.

Accreditation challenges make it critical that the library designate a point person to lead accreditation efforts. This person will be the library point person for stakeholders as the accreditation process for the organization evolves. This person will also attend all planning meetings and keep the rest of the library apprised of any new developments. It is not critical that this person be a library administrator. Those in library administration have many different responsibilities and may not have the time to engage in this process fully. Choosing a point person who is not a library administrator may benefit the library more because the person will have time to devote to the process. In addition, the person may have better relationships with those involved, which may facilitate better communication with stakeholders. Regardless of who is chosen to lead library efforts, the person selected needs to have a complete understanding of accreditation standards. This understanding will be important as this person develops a work plan with library staff. This work plan will lay out a timeline that lists key tasks and dates, which will help library staff better understand the process and what will be required.

Upon reviewing these standards, an organization will do a self-assessment based on these standards to identify gaps or deficiencies in the organization's procedures, structures, processes, and policies. Those going through accreditation tend to adopt continuous quality improvement (CQI) processes to effectively identify and address these gaps.[29,30,31,32] CQI is a process that a library participating in accreditation activities should also adopt. It will allow a library to be a continual learning organization that can identify issues early and put a process in place to address them. CQI is where an organization constantly looks to improve what is being done. Those in these organizations ask questions like "How are we doing?" or "What can be done to do it better or be more effective?"[33] The CQI process is where an organization or group goes through a series of continual plan, do, study, act (PDSA) cycles. This cycle starts with the planning stage (P), where a problem is identified, and a plan is made to address the problem. The next step is to do (D). During this step, an intervention is implemented to address the identified issue. Once the intervention has been implemented for a period of time, then the effectiveness of the process must be studied (S) to determine if the intervention is addressing the issue effectively. The effectiveness of the intervention is determined by a set of predetermined measures or benchmarks. These criteria should be based on the accreditation standards. If the intervention is effective, the process moves forward to act (A) and adopts this intervention as the standard for the organization. Regardless of whether the desired outcome is achieved or not, the cycle starts again. There is always some improvement that can be made, so the process is continual.[34,35] To ensure the gains are maintained, mechanisms must be put in place to gather the data necessary to track effectiveness. The data needed in the accreditation process may already be gathered as it may be required for annual reports to the American Library Association (ALA), Association of College & Research Libraries (ACRL), Association of Academic Health Sciences Libraries (AAHSL), or other organizations. Any gaps in the data gathered or policies needed to support the accreditation process must be addressed.

YEAR 2: MONITORING PROGRESS AND MAKING ADJUSTMENTS

During the second year of the accreditation process, the organization and library should be engaged in continuing to improve to meet all aspects of the accreditation standards. In this second year, the library should ensure that communication with the stakeholders going through accreditation is continual and that regular check-ins are established to ensure that library efforts continue to be aligned with the organization's efforts.

Not only should the library have regular communication with stakeholders outside of the library, but library administrators must remember to be in regular communication with library staff. It should be clear to library staff where the library fits in the process, the expectations for each team member, and the timeline for the accreditation process. During this time, it is crucial to make sure that all involved staff members in the library are aware of any self-study activities that the library has or will be doing. This awareness will help library staff to buy into the process. It will also be essential to highlight any findings from the self-assessment to identify potential solutions to address weaknesses and increase organizational pride by highlighting the library's strengths.

Communication should be bidirectional with stakeholders and library staff. Bidirectional communication is where information flows both ways. Good communication is key to successful CQI activities, especially when it comes to managing the expectations and addressing the concerns of stakeholders and library staff. Clear communication is critical if the library cannot meet some aspects of the expectations placed on the library by stakeholders or accreditation standards. The library must be clear about what is achievable and not achievable to prevent any last-minute surprises and maintain a good relationship with stakeholders.

YEAR 3: PREPARING PRELIMINARY REPORT & CONTINUING ACTIVITIES TO MEET ACCREDITATION STANDARDS

In the third year of the accreditation cycle, stakeholders focus on preparing a preliminary report. The report submitted to the accreditation organization is a self-report prepared by the organization that provides data and other supporting evidence to demonstrate how the organization is meeting the standards for accreditation. During the creation of this report, the library may be asked for data and evidence that support the accreditation standards. The library collection and resources provided to support learning may be mentioned in the report. At other times, the library may be asked to assist in developing a part of the report that may mention library services or activities that an organization believes are notable in meeting accreditation standards.

Submission of the report does not mean the organization or the library is done with accreditation. There is always room to improve, and any improvement plans continue along with the data collection that supports it.

YEAR 4: PREPARING AND PARTICIPATING IN THE SITE VISIT

The fourth year of the accreditation cycle is the culmination of the organization's and the library's efforts. It is when the organization will make final adjustments to its procedures, structures, processes, and policies to ensure they are in line with accreditation standards. During this year, these adjustments and planning are focused on for the site visit. An on-site team conducts this visit for between one and three days. The main purpose of this visit is to verify that the items in the self-report are being implemented and accreditation standards are being met. A secondary goal for these visits is to identify how well the organization is doing. The amplification of the good things going on in the organization is a time when library services or involvement may be recognized.

To be recognized, the library needs to have a part in planning the visit. The organization is notified a couple of months in advance about site visits. To ensure that the library is prepared, the library needs to be in contact with stakeholders and attend any preparation meetings when possible. The schedule for the visit will be key to the library being able to participate effectively and understand what the expectations will be during the visit. For example, the library may be asked to present to the accreditation team activities related to the standards. These presentations are essential and will take preparation. The library may also be asked

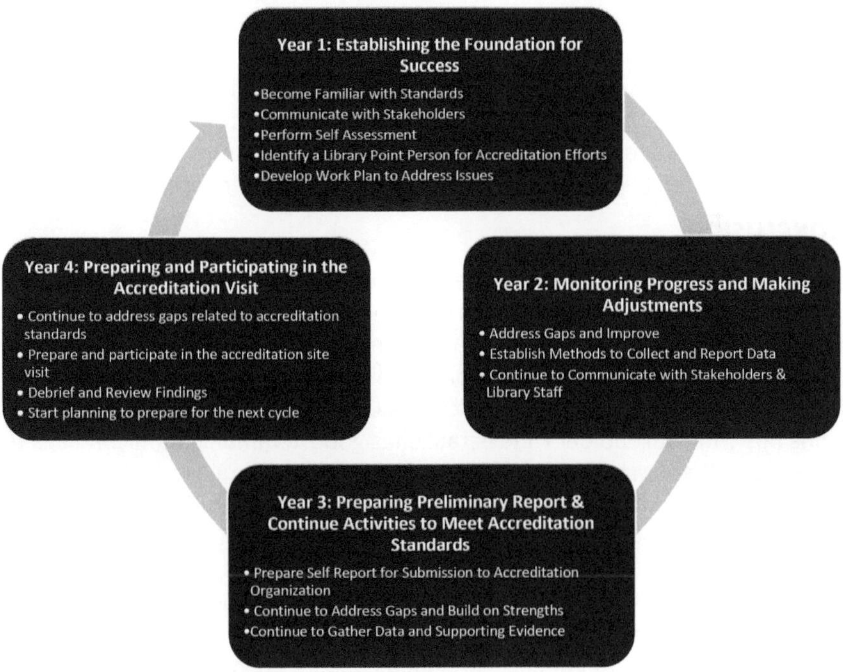

Figure 2.1. The Accreditation Cycle (4-Year Cycle)
SOURCE: ROY BROWN

to discuss library collections or resources that support clinical or educational programs. A library tour may also be requested.

Most site visits will end with a debriefing session with the site visit team, where the team provides some insight into their initial findings and discusses the next steps. These next steps will include when the final report will be submitted and when a final accreditation decision will be made. During this debriefing session, the team may also take some questions, but the time for this will likely be limited. The debriefing session with the site visit team should be the first of several sessions. The organization's stakeholders should hold the next session within days of the site visit. This session will discuss observations about what went well, what did not go so well, and some initial impressions based on interactions by those involved in the visit both in and outside of the library. An additional session may be necessary once the final report and decision on accreditation are received. This final report will provide clear areas for improvement and highlight the organization's strengths.

Regardless of how many meetings or debriefing sessions are held once the site visit is over, it must be noted that receiving accreditation is not the end of the road. Accreditation is intended to be cyclical and forces organizations to participate in continually reflecting on what is being done and how it can be improved. This continual reflection means that the sooner a library starts to focus on the next accreditation cycle, the better positioned the library will be to support the stakeholders going through the process the next time. The continual nature of accreditation means it is vital to keep communication channels with stakeholders open; staying apprised of any changes in accreditation standards is critical. Accreditation standards are not static but are constantly reevaluated and adjusted to reflect changes in the healthcare environment (see figure 2.1).

CONCLUSION

Accreditation is a key driver of change in health professions' education and patient care. While the role of libraries in meeting accreditation standards is not always clear, it is important to understand the process and figure out how to best support stakeholders as they go through accreditation. Supporting the process will only be possible if the library forges good relationships with stakeholders and establishes good communication channels to understand the library's expectations. It will benefit the library to understand the particular accreditation standards and identify opportunities to contribute that those stakeholders may not recognize. Regardless of the extent to which libraries are involved in the accreditation process, it is a critical way that a library can show value to an organization. Libraries must be thoughtful in addressing the process and start planning sooner rather than later. One way to ensure success is to adopt a continuous quality improvement approach to addressing problems within the library. The library should continually assess strengths and weaknesses and make plans to improve based on the data collected. Adopting a CQI mindset ensures the library is constantly evolving, stays agile, and can meet the needs of stakeholders going through an accreditation cycle. Utilizing the CQI process requires a clear plan and time to devote to the process. A clear, timely plan is crucial for libraries regarding accreditation. To best meet accreditation challenges and demonstrate value, a library needs a point person and a clear plan. This plan allows a library to best prepare for accreditation and be successful.

NOTES

1. Hema N. Viswanathan and J. Warren Salmon, "Accrediting Organizations and Quality Improvement," *American Journal of Managed Care* 6, no. 10 (2000): 1117–30.

2. Tom Schmiedel, "Library Support for Accreditation: A Guide to Online Resources," *College and Research Libraries News* 78, no. 2 (2017): 96–100, https://doi.org/10.5860/crln.78.2.9624.

3. Michele R. Tennant et al., "Information and Scientific Literacy Support Aligning Instruction with Standards and Frames to Prepare Students for Research and Lifelong Learning," in *The New Information Literacy Instruction: Best Practices*, ed. Patrick Ragains and M. Sandra Wood (Lanham, MD: Rowman & Littlefield, 2015), 137–52.

4. Tessa Withorn et al., "Library Instruction and Information Literacy 2020," *Reference Services Review* 49, no. 3-4 (2021): 329–418, https://doi.org/10.1108/RSR-07-2021-0046.

5. Riley Brian et al., "Evaluating the Impact of Clinical Librarians on Clinical Questions during Inpatient Rounds," *Journal of the Medical Library Association: JMLA* 106, no. 2 (April 2018): 175–83, https://doi.org/10.5195/JMLA.2018.254.

6. Julia M. Esparza et al., "The Effect of a Clinical Medical Librarian on In-Patient Care Outcomes," *Journal of the Medical Library Association: JMLA* 101, no. 3 (2013): 185–91, https://doi.org/10.3163/1536-5050.101.3.007.

7. Pamela Hargwood and Christopher Duffy, "Out of the Library and on to the Floors: Librarian Participation in Nursing Rounds," *Journal of Hospital Librarianship* 16, no. 3 (2016): 209–14.

8. Kay Cimpl Wagner and Gary D. Byrd, "Evaluating the Effectiveness of Clinical Medical Librarian Programs: A Systematic Review of the Literature," *Journal of the Medical Library Association* 92, no. 1 (2004): 14–33.

9. Roy E. Brown, "Empowering Nurses with an Online Roadmap for Evidence-Based Practice," *Journal of Hospital Librarianship* 20, no. 4 (October 2020): 309–22, https://doi.org/10.1080/15323269.2020.1819748.

10. Kerry Dhakal, "Librarians Collaborating to Teach Evidence-Based Practice: Exploring Partnerships with Professional Organizations," *Journal of the Medical Library Association: JMLA* 106, no. 3 (July 2018): 311–19, https://doi.org/10.5195/JMLA.2018.341.

11. Zachary R. Krom, Janene Batten, and Cynthia Bautista, "A Unique Collaborative Nursing Evidence-Based Practice Initiative Using the Iowa Model: A Clinical Nurse Specialist, a Health Science Librarian, and a Staff Nurse's Success Story," *Clinical Nurse Specialist CNS* 24, no. 2 (March 2010): 54–59, https://doi.org/10.1097/NUR.0B013E3181CF5537.

12. Lauren A. Maggio, Nancy Durieux, and Nancy H. Tannery, "Librarians in Evidence-Based Medicine Curricula: A Qualitative Study of Librarian Roles, Training, and Desires for Future Development," *Medical Reference Services Quarterly* 34, no. 4 (October 2015): 428–40, https://doi.org/10.1080/02763869.2015.1082375.
13. Connie Schardt, "Evidence-Based Medicine and the Hospital Librarian," *Journal of Hospital Librarianship* 1, no. 2 (2001): 1–14.
14. Christine Willis, Kate Daniels, and Margaret Gettis, "A Collaborative Effort to Build an Evidence-Based Practice Project Repository," *Medical Reference Services Quarterly* 40, no. 2 (2021): 205–14.
15. Christine A. Willis, "Hospital Accreditation: A Primer," *Journal of Hospital Librarianship* 21, no. 3 (2021): 289–99, https://doi.org/10.1080/15323269.2021.1967685.
16. US Centers for Medicare & Medicaid Services, "Centers for Medicare & Medicaid Services," 2022, https://www.cms.gov/.
17. US Centers for Medicare & Medicaid Services, "CMS Strategic Plan," April 2022, https://www.cms.gov/cms-strategic-plan.
18. US Centers for Medicare & Medicaid Services, "Quality Improvement Organizations," December 2021, https://www.cms.gov/Medicare/Quality-Initiatives-Patient-Assessment-Instruments/QualityImprovementOrgs.
19. Miranda B. Lam et al., "Association between Patient Outcomes and Accreditation in US Hospitals: Observational Study," *BMJ (Online)* 363 (2018), https://doi.org/10.1136/bmj.k4011.
20. Lam et al., "Patient Outcomes and Accreditation."
21. Jafar S. Tabrizi, Farid Gharibi, and Andrew J. Wilson, "Advantages and Disadvantages of Health Care Accreditation," *Health Promotion Perspectives* 1, no. 1 (2011): 1–31, https://doi.org/10.5681/HPP.2011.001.
22. Jonathan D. Eldredge et al., "Current Practices in Library/Informatics Instruction in Academic Libraries Serving Medical Schools in the Western United States: A Three-Phase Action Research Study," *BMC Medical Education* 13, no. 1 (2013), https://doi.org/10.1186/1472-6920-13-119.
23. Mark MacEachern et al., "Librarian Integration in a Four-Year Medical School Curriculum: A Timeline," *Medical Reference Services Quarterly* 31, no. 1 (January 2012): 105–14, https://doi.org/10.1080/02763869.2012.641856.
24. Amanda M. Nevius et al., "Library Instruction in Medical Education: A Survey of Current Practices in the United States and Canada," *Journal of the Medical Library Association: JMLA* 106, no. 1 (January 2018): 98–98, https://doi.org/10.5195/JMLA.2018.374.
25. Commission on the Accreditation of Rehabilitation Facilities, "CARF International," 2022, http://www.carf.org/home/.
26. American Nurses Credentialing Center, "About Magnet," 2022, https://www.nursingworld.org/organizational-programs/magnet/about-magnet/.
27. American Association of Colleges of Nursing, "Vizient/AACN Nurse Residency Program," 2022, https://www.aacnnursing.org/nurse-residency-program.
28. The Joint Commission, "The Unannounced Survey Process," 2022, https://www.jointcommission.org/-/media/08c0024441f54848b8c212dd0b5dbeff.ashx.
29. Barbara Barzansky et al., "Continuous Quality Improvement in an Accreditation System for Undergraduate Medical Education: Benefits and Challenges," *Medical Teacher* 37, no. 11 (November 2015): 1032–38, https://doi.org/10.3109/0142159X.2015.1031735.

30. Nesibe Akdemir et al., "Evaluation of Continuous Quality Improvement in Accreditation for Medical Education," *BMC Medical Education* 20 (September 2020), https://doi.org/10.1186/s12909-020-02124-2.
31. Peggy Ellis and Judith Halstead, "Understanding the Commission on Collegiate Nursing Education Accreditation Process and the Role of the Continuous Improvement Progress Report," *Journal of Professional Nursing* 28, no. 1 (January 2012): 18–26, https://doi.org/10.1016/j.profnurs.2011.10.004.
32. Ellie Scrivens, "Putting Continuous Quality Improvement into Accreditation: Improving Approaches to Quality Assessment," *Quality and Safety in Health Care* 6, no. 4 (1997): 212–18, https://doi.org/10.1136/qshc.6.4.212.
33. US Department of Health and Human Services, "Continuous Quality Improvement (CQI) Strategies to Optimize Your Practice," 2013.
34. Agency for Healthcare Research and Quality, "Plan-Do-Study-Act (PDSA) Directions and Examples | Agency for Healthcare Research and Quality," September 2020, https://www.ahrq.gov/health-literacy/improve/precautions/tool2b.html.
35. B. O'Donnell and V. Gupta, "Continuous Quality Improvement," in *StatPearls*, 2022, https://www.ncbi.nlm.nih.gov/books/NBK559239/.

BIBLIOGRAPHY

Agency for Healthcare Research and Quality. "Plan-Do-Study-Act (PDSA) Directions and Examples | Agency for Healthcare Research and Quality." September 2020. https://www.ahrq.gov/health-literacy/improve/precautions/tool2b.html.

Aitken, Elizabeth M., Susan E. Powelson, Renée D. Reaume, and William A. Ghali. "Involving Clinical Librarians at the Point of Care: Results of a Controlled Intervention." *Academic Medicine* 86, no. 12 (2011): 1508–12. https://doi.org/10.1097/ACM.0b013e31823595cd.

Akdemir, Nesibe, Linda N. Peterson, Craig M. Campbell, and Fedde Scheele. "Evaluation of Continuous Quality Improvement in Accreditation for Medical Education." *BMC Medical Education* 20 (September 2020). https://doi.org/10.1186/s12909-020-02124-2.

American Association of Colleges of Nursing. "Vizient/AACN Nurse Residency Program," 2022. https://www.aacnnursing.org/nurse-residency-program.

American Nurses Credentialing Center. "About Magnet," 2022. https://www.nursingworld.org/organizational-programs/magnet/about-magnet/.

Barzansky, Barbara, Dan Hunt, Geneviève Moineau, Ducksun Ahn, Chi Wan Lai, Holly Humphrey, and Linda Peterson. "Continuous Quality Improvement in an Accreditation System for Undergraduate Medical Education: Benefits and Challenges." *Medical Teacher* 37, no. 11 (November 2015): 1032–38. https://doi.org/10.3109/0142159X.2015.1031735.

Blouin, Danielle, and Ara Tekian. "Accreditation of Medical Education Programs: Moving from Student Outcomes to Continuous Quality Improvement Measures." *Academic Medicine* 93, no. 3 (2018): 377–83. https://doi.org/10.1097/ACM.0000000000001835.

Brian, Riley, Nicola Orlov, Debra Werner, Shannon K. Martin, Vineet M. Arora, and Maria Alkureishi. "Evaluating the Impact of Clinical Librarians on Clinical Questions during Inpatient Rounds." *Journal of the Medical Library Association: JMLA* 106, no. 2 (April 2018): 175–83. https://doi.org/10.5195/JMLA.2018.254.

Brown, Roy E. "Empowering Nurses with an Online Roadmap for Evidence-Based Practice." *Journal of Hospital Librarianship* 20, no. 4 (October 2020): 309–22. https://doi.org/10.1080/15323269.2020.1819748.

Commission on the Accreditation of Rehabilitation Facilities. "CARF International," 2022. http://www.carf.org/home/.

Dhakal, Kerry. "Librarians Collaborating to Teach Evidence-Based Practice: Exploring Partnerships with Professional Organizations." *Journal of the Medical Library Association: JMLA* 106, no. 3 (July 2018): 311–19. https://doi.org/10.5195/JMLA.2018.341.

Eldredge, Jonathan D., Karen M. Heskett, Terry Henner, and Josephine P. Tan. "Current Practices in Library/Informatics Instruction in Academic Libraries Serving Medical Schools in the Western United States: A Three-Phase Action Research Study." *BMC Medical Education* 13, no. 1 (2013). https://doi.org/10.1186/1472-6920-13-119.

Ellis, Peggy, and Judith Halstead. "Understanding the Commission on Collegiate Nursing Education Accreditation Process and the Role of the Continuous Improvement Progress Report." *Journal of Professional Nursing* 28, no. 1 (January 2012): 18–26. https://doi.org/10.1016/j.profnurs.2011.10.004.

Esparza, Julia M., Runhua Shi, Jerry McLarty, Marianne Comegys, and Daniel E. Banks. "The Effect of a Clinical Medical Librarian on In-Patient Care Outcomes." *Journal of the Medical Library Association: JMLA* 101, no. 3 (2013): 185–91. https://doi.org/10.3163/1536-5050.101.3.007.

Hargwood, Pamela, and Christopher Duffy. "Out of the Library and on to the Floors: Librarian Participation in Nursing Rounds." *Journal of Hospital Librarianship* 16, no. 3 (2016): 209–14.

Joint Commission. "The Unannounced Survey Process," 2022. https://www.jointcommission.org/-/media/08c0024441f54848b8c212dd0b5dbeff.ashx.

Krom, Zachary R., Janene Batten, and Cynthia Bautista. "A Unique Collaborative Nursing Evidence-Based Practice Initiative Using the Iowa Model: A Clinical Nurse Specialist, a Health Science Librarian, and a Staff Nurse's Success Story." *Clinical Nurse Specialist CNS* 24, no. 2 (March 2010): 54–59. https://doi.org/10.1097/NUR.0B013E3181CF5537.

Lam, Miranda B., Jose F. Figueroa, Yevgeniy Feyman, Kimberly E. Reimold, E. John Orav, and Ashish K. Jha. "Association between Patient Outcomes and Accreditation in US Hospitals: Observational Study." *BMJ (Online)* 363 (2018). https://doi.org/10.1136/bmj.k4011.

MacEachern, Mark, Whitney Townsend, Kristen Young, and Gurpreet Rana. "Librarian Integration in a Four-Year Medical School Curriculum: A Timeline." *Medical Reference Services Quarterly* 31, no. 1 (January 2012): 105–14. https://doi.org/10.1080/02763869.2012.641856.

Maggio, Lauren A., Nancy Durieux, and Nancy H. Tannery. "Librarians in Evidence-Based Medicine Curricula: A Qualitative Study of Librarian Roles, Training, and Desires for Future Development." *Medical Reference Services Quarterly* 34, no. 4 (October 2015): 428–40. https://doi.org/10.1080/02763869.2015.1082375.

Nevius, Amanda M., A'Llyn Ettien, Alissa P. Link, and Laura Y. Sobel. "Library Instruction in Medical Education: A Survey of Current Practices in the United States and Canada." *Journal of the Medical Library Association: JMLA* 106, no. 1 (January 2018): 98–98. https://doi.org/10.5195/JMLA.2018.374.

O'Donnell, B., and V. Gupta. "Continuous Quality Improvement." In *StatPearls*, 2022. https://www.ncbi.nlm.nih.gov/books/NBK559239/.

Schardt, Connie. "Evidence-Based Medicine and the Hospital Librarian." *Journal of Hospital Librarianship* 1, no. 2 (2001): 1–14.

Schmiedel, Tom. "Library Support for Accreditation: A Guide to Online Resources." *College and Research Libraries News* 78, no. 2 (2017): 96–100. https://doi.org/10.5860/crln.78.2.9624.

Scrivens, Ellie. "Putting Continuous Quality Improvement into Accreditation: Improving Approaches to Quality Assessment." *Quality and Safety in Health Care* 6, no. 4 (1997): 212–18. https://doi.org/10.1136/qshc.6.4.212.

Tabrizi, Jafar S., Farid Gharibi, and Andrew J. Wilson. "Advantages and Disadvantages of Health Care Accreditation Models." *Health Promotion Perspectives* 1, no. 1 (2011): 1–31. https://doi.org/10.5681/HPP.2011.001.

Tennant, Michele R., Mary E. Edwards, Hannah F. Norton, and Sara Russell Gonzalez. "Information and Scientific Literacy Support Aligning Instruction with Standards and Frames to Prepare Students for Research and Lifelong Learning." In *New Information Literacy Instruction: Best Practices*, edited by Patrick Ragains and M. Sandra Wood, 137–52. Lanham, MD: Rowman & Littlefield, 2015.

US Centers for Medicare & Medicaid Services. "Centers for Medicare & Medicaid Services," 2022. https://www.cms.gov/.

———. "CMS Strategic Plan," April 2022. https://www.cms.gov/cms-strategic-plan.

———. "Quality Improvement Organizations," December 2021. https://www.cms.gov/Medicare/Quality-Initiatives-Patient-Assessment-Instruments/QualityImprovementOrgs.

US Department of Health and Human Services. "Continuous Quality Improvement (CQI) Strategies to Optimize Your Practice," 2013.

Viswanathan, Hema N., and J. Warren Salmon. "Accrediting Organizations and Quality Improvement." *American Journal of Managed Care* 6, no. 10 (2000): 1117–30.

Wagner, Kay Cimpl, and Gary D. Byrd. "Evaluating the Effectiveness of Clinical Medical Librarian Programs: A Systematic Review of the Literature." *Journal of the Medical Library Association* 92, no. 1 (2004): 14–33.

Willis, Christine A. "Hospital Accreditation: A Primer." *Journal of Hospital Librarianship* 21, no. 3 (2021): 289–99. https://doi.org/10.1080/15323269.2021.1967685.

Willis, Christine, Kate Daniels, and Margaret Gettis. "A Collaborative Effort to Build an Evidence-Based Practice Project Repository." *Medical Reference Services Quarterly* 40, no. 2 (2021): 205–14.

Withorn, Tessa, Jillian Eslami, Hannah Lee, Maggie Clarke, Carolyn Caffrey Gardner, Cristina Springfield, Dana Ospina, et al. "Library Instruction and Information Literacy 2020." *Reference Services Review* 49, no. 3–4 (2021): 329–418. https://doi.org/10.1108/RSR-07-2021-0046.

3

Maintaining Continuity through Personnel Changes

Ana Corral and Rachel Helbing, University of Houston

Despite their reputation for rigidity, libraries, and health sciences libraries in particular, are constantly being reshaped and restructured, adapting to the needs of their users, institutions, and the communities they serve.[1] While these transformations can arise from shifts in technology or research needs, institutional recalibration is often accompanied by personnel changes, which in turn can affect the flow of institutional knowledge and continuity of plans. The fragmentation of shared knowledge can erode professional relationships and procedures, resulting in departmental silos and fractured communication. This splintering can become especially problematic when a health sciences library provides support during an accreditation process. The relationship between a health sciences library and the health professions programs it supports, and the critical needs that librarians address during this process, are significant. This is especially true if the accreditation is for a newly established program that is relying on a successful outcome. In this chapter, the authors will draw upon their experiences supporting the University of Houston's new community-focused College of Medicine as they navigate the Liaison Committee on Medical Education (LCME) accreditation process while simultaneously experiencing personnel changes and library growth. The authors will discuss how to utilize best practices in forming strategic partnerships, maintaining open lines of communication, and the sharing and recording of institutional knowledge and how these approaches can best support a successful accreditation process.

BEST PRACTICES FOR ACCREDITATION DURING INSTITUTIONAL GROWTH AND TRANSITION

Institutions of higher education have undergone significant changes in the twenty-first century.[2] Technological advances have altered the way students interact with information and each other and how instructional material is disseminated and consumed. More and more courses and programs of higher education are transitioning to online modalities or offering hybrid alternatives, bringing to light growing pains and unanticipated modifications in how instructors engage with both students and their fields of expertise. The growing reach of technology comes along with adjustments in research focus. The University of Houston, a recently designated Carnegie 1 Research Institution, has had to reassess, revamp, and revise its output, approach, and engagement with research capacity. The institution is quickly pivoting to remain competitive and up to date with the technological and research advancements of institutions of higher education in the United States by implementing two new programs. First is 50-in-5,[3] an initiative to increase research output by 50 percent in five years. Next is the new Presidential Frontiers Faculty[4] program, designed to grow interdisciplinary development in key research areas. These two programs, coupled with the University of Houston's ambitious new strategic plan, demonstrate a growing commitment and new focus on transformative research topics, intentional engagement, and innovative technology.

While academic libraries are experiencing their own recalibration and expansion, they are also guided and influenced by the development of the institutions with which they are affiliated. These transformations often take tangible shape in strategic plans, reassessment of mission statements, goals, and core values, the expansion of new, innovative departments, and the restructuring or removal of outdated areas of focus or positions. While these changes are signs of positive growth for the institutions and their libraries, they can also leave library personnel feeling uncertain, stressed, and anxious about their roles within their libraries and the broader institutions of which they are a part.[5] These changes can also impact the way librarians engage with and support their liaison areas and the broader university community. Shifting university and library priorities and strategic areas of focus that have been previously established can cause lack of clarity and understanding of library objectives and liaison goals, forcing health sciences librarians to make modifications for which they may not be prepared.

While these growing pains are a part of every academic librarian's experience, they can cause a variance in levels and capacity of engagement with students and liaison areas. They are a part of everyday life, yet the accreditation process stops for no one. Achieving and maintaining LCME accreditation can be a lengthy and meticulous process, requiring long-term vision and commitment to maintain LCME standards, which again can be greatly impacted by varying goals and values of the institution and affiliated library. As such, health sciences librarians must be nimble and adaptive as they navigate these various responsibilities. To help support this, librarians can employ several intentional strategies such as strategic engagement, maintaining continuity, communicating effectively, and utilizing key resources at their disposal.

STRATEGIC ENGAGEMENT—WITHIN THE LIBRARIES

To successfully assist in an accreditation process for a newly established school, it is imperative that the health sciences librarian supporting the process be intimately familiar with both the needs of the medical school and the areas of the library that can best provide support and resources during the process. If a health sciences librarian is new in their role or if there has been institutional recalibration and restructuring, a mitigating approach can be taken through strategic engagement of the stakeholders in their library who will play a role in the accreditation process. Identifying the library divisions that need to be involved will ensure that the accreditation process, which for the LCME includes a data collection instrument (DCI), independent student analysis (ISA), and site visit, will go smoothly. First, educating themselves on the needs of the current accreditation level a medical school has is critical; they might have to rely on the institutional knowledge of one specific department more heavily than another to support the medical school during the process. Certain parts of the LCME accreditation process, such as during the site visit or the DCI, call for specific information about library resources, physical spaces, electronic and physical access, and number of personnel—information that informs the LCME on how well the library is equipped to support the new program.[6] Divisions or departments in the library that manage collections, electronic access, physical spaces, and health sciences services are essential in providing information, infrastructure, and resources needed for the accreditation process.

While a health sciences librarian does not need to be an expert in all these library areas, identifying and connecting with these divisions is indispensable to the success of the report writing and the site visit. The needs of the LCME site visit team and the medical school can also vary depending on the type of LCME application (e.g., preliminary accreditation or provisional accreditation); as such, reassessing which divisions you need to be in communication with is warranted. Staying in contact and informed through strategic and targeted engagement of these divisions will both help the accreditation process and aid in documentation that will be needed during the next step in the accreditation journey of the program and to maintain LCME standards.

STRATEGIC ENGAGEMENT—WITH THE MEDICAL SCHOOL

Maintaining engagement for accreditation success extends beyond the libraries to the medical school that is actively going through an accreditation process. Strategically connecting the work that a medical school is doing to the support and services provided by their health sciences librarian is paramount to meet the ongoing LCME standards of accreditation. It is important to find synergies between the program and the library and to make sure they are aligned with the standards of the LCME. Identifying essential team members, such as the office of medical education, the office of graduate education, and the office of assessment and quality improvement, and arranging strategic meetings, partnerships, and joint tasks as needed will also aid in the accreditation process.

While some solo librarians and smaller libraries might grapple with their capacity to support a medical school during the accreditation process and to maintain high participation in liaison duties and other professional commitments, engaging in a way that the medical school most needs requires transparency, communication, and flexibility. One medical school might need its health sciences librarian present only during the site visit or to provide particulars during the information-gathering part of the report, while another may ask for a more embedded role. The University of Houston's College of Medicine took the latter route when it asked its health sciences librarian to serve as a liaison to the ISA committee.

As stated by the Association of American Medical Colleges (AAMC),

> The goal of this Independent Student Analysis is to generate student feedback in order to illustrate the strengths and weaknesses of each medical school, measured in comparison to multiple standards that the LCME outlines. The ISA is a student project and should be treated as such by not only the students, but the faculty and administration as well. Thus, it is important for students to take the lead and not allow any distortion or misrepresentation of the data by faculty or administration.[7]

Given that the report cannot be influenced or interfered upon by the medical school or any faculty member, the aim of having a health sciences librarian liaise with the student committee is to provide resources related to conducting a survey and the survey process and serve as a resource of whom they could ask process support and confidential questions. They could safely do this with no influence, intervention, or impact upon the survey, the data collection, and the resulting recommendations. Liaising with the ISA committee, to whatever extent possible and if the invitation is extended, can provide liaisons and other library personnel a better understanding of the critical role that the ISA committee and resulting recommendations have upon the accreditation process. By serving as a resource throughout the process of the survey, resulting recommendations, and the site visit, health sciences librarians can position themselves as partners and key players in the success of the accreditation process.

Last, smaller libraries that do not have the capacity for fully embedded engagement approaches can participate in committees and subcommittees in the medical school. As Wood tells us, "Medical librarians have a long history of service on college-level curriculum committees," an experience that benefits both the library and the medical school as it creates a collaborative experience with its health sciences librarian and fosters "a partnership that provides information assistance to clients, [and] keeps committee members apprised of resources and services available in the library."[8] Attending and participating on curricular committees, including subcommittees that overview the maintenance of accreditation, can simultaneously benefit both the medical school and the librarian, fostering the ability for health sciences librarians to showcase their information literacy skills and the services and support they can provide while also providing a richer understanding of how medical education is created, modified, and supported by faculty, staff, and administration.

BEST PRACTICES DURING PERSONNEL CHANGES

Career mobility among all workers, including librarians, is growing. Rather than staying at one library for the entirety of their careers, many will move between different institutions and geographic regions multiple times in their professional lives. As of January 2020, the median employee tenure was 4.1 years, according to the US Bureau of Labor Statistics.[9] This employee movement is often positive in that it can facilitate the influx of new ideas and bring growth to both the professionals and their organizations. At the same time, frequent turnover can make it difficult to maintain continuity during wide-scale longitudinal projects such as achieving accreditation for new health professions programs. Having practices in place to minimize the amount of institutional knowledge lost when someone leaves a key position in the library or the academic unit can make a tangible difference to the ability to successfully attain accreditation.

HOW TO MAINTAIN CONTINUITY OF PLANS

An important consideration for maintaining continuity during an accreditation process is to not rely on a single person to manage the library's involvement. If there is an individual controlling all accreditation documents and relationships, it could be catastrophic if that person were to leave the institution, be unavailable for another reason, or even have a technology failure. Making sure that multiple people in the library are fully apprised of the accreditation process and requirements is necessary. In line with this, it is recommended to utilize simple technological tools like shared online documents. If there are any personnel disruptions, other library staff with access to the documents can step in and build on the progress that has already been made. When turnover does happen, it is necessary to conduct a meaningful information-sharing session with any exiting employee who has been involved in the accreditation process, to ensure no documents, details, or deadlines are missed.

HOW TO MAINTAIN FLOW OF INSTITUTIONAL KNOWLEDGE

Clear documentation is key to maintaining the flow of institutional knowledge through personnel changes. Expanding on the suggestion to utilize shared documents, one way to achieve this is by curating a knowledge base of documents related to accreditation. At the University of Houston, the Health Sciences

Library supports five health sciences colleges as well as additional health sciences programs housed in other colleges. Librarians are frequently asked to provide a letter or narrative and/or fill out a questionnaire providing detailed information about the library's collections and services in order to support these various health sciences programs' accreditation or grant applications. The information requested can include the size of the print and electronic collections, notable journal subscriptions, square footage of the physical space and available seating, number of professional staff, research support services provided, and more. While each request is different and must be individualized for that program, much of the information is the same and can be reused. Keeping these documents in a knowledge base that is easily accessible to all library staff can save time and effort spent on re-creating similar requests and provide a historical record of requests. The record can be used to identify the accreditation cycles of relevant programs and create a calendar of due dates in order to be prepared for requests. It can also be used as an onboarding tool. New hires can skim through past requests to get a sense of the ways that the library supports different programs as well as the programs' accreditation requirements. They can also build off past documents when fulfilling requests. Additionally, analysis of the knowledge base can make it easier to identify gaps in library services being offered between programs.

Another type of accreditation documentation to maintain in the library is a list of contacts. Each program will typically have an individual who is ultimately responsible for the accreditation application and associated site visit. There may also be a separate individual who is assigned to take the lead on the document needing input and collaboration from the library. Maintaining a list of these contacts that can be passed on to any new library staff will help to keep the process on track. Additionally, if a person from the list leaves, the library can proactively reach out to their replacement to establish contact. This will help ensure that the library stays involved in the accreditation process regardless of personnel turnover in the library or the program.

COMMUNICATION—TARGETED AND TRANSPARENT

Ultimately, one of the best practices health sciences librarians can employ is communicating their capacity and any time constraints they may be experiencing. The journey toward accreditation involves many key players in both the health sciences library and the medical school itself. Effective teamwork and collaboration require transparent communication—about how much support health sciences librarians can realistically provide and what services the library as a whole can provide and support. Academic librarians have reported experiencing burnout, fatigue caused by workplace stress that can manifest itself both mentally and physically, to some extent since library-focused research first began to be conducted on the topic in the late 1990s.[10] While burnout is impacted by numerous factors such as toxic work conditions, microaggressions, and unhealthy work-life balance, being overworked can also have a huge impact. Burnout is a part of the academic world that health sciences librarians navigate, and this is something that librarians working alone or in a smaller library with fewer resources to support an accreditation process need to consider. Being clear about capacity is crucial, not just to the professional and personal well-being of the health sciences librarians involved but also to the accreditation process itself. It is vital to be conscious about how much support and service a health sciences librarian can provide as compared to the needs and expectations of the medical school during their accreditation process. The need to be forthright and transparent about the time commitment required during accreditation, especially during preparations for and during site visits, must be clearly communicated among the entire accreditation team. Transparent communication about the expected contribution and effort also extends to the library team of which the health sciences librarian is a part. From allocating time to gather information for the report to reviewing previous site visits with predecessors to preparing the health sciences librarian and the library during mock site visits: all require transparency and care. Communicating abilities and time constraints is a necessity.

UTILIZING RESOURCES

When working through an accreditation process, it is important to remember that you are not the first librarian to chart these waters. There is support available from colleagues who have been through this before. This can come both through formal channels, such as continuing education and professional organization resources, and informal channels, such as unofficial mentoring relationships.

Look for continuing education opportunities from within librarianship and from the field in which accreditation is being sought. Library organizations to consult include the Medical Library Association (MLA) and the Association of Academic Health Sciences Libraries (AAHSL). Both offer coursework, workshops, and conferences that can provide insight into and detailed advice on accreditation processes. Within medical education, the Association of American Medical Colleges (AAMC) hosts relevant webinars and conferences, especially those that specifically cover the LCME accreditation process. The LCME website also provides a plethora of checklists, standards, and processes that can be mined and utilized.

Another source of potential support is the existing knowledge in the institution. Again, documentation is key; LCME documents from prior accreditation rounds can be invaluable moving forward. Additionally, seek out faculty and/or librarian mentors. Identify opportunities for cross-training with librarian colleagues who have worked on accreditation projects in the past. At small or solo libraries, however, these resources may not exist, and it is perfectly acceptable to do what can feasibly be done and rely on the experts in the academic program as needed.

Finally, utilize informal sources of support in professional organizations and in the medical librarian field generally. Organization listservs contain a wealth of wisdom, both current and historical. It is prudent to search the listserv archives to check if a particular issue has already been addressed and then, if needed, send a message to the list to seek updated responses or begin a conversation on a previously unaddressed topic. Additionally, professional organizations may include interest groups or committees on accreditation-related topics. For example, AAHSL has a New and Developing Health Sciences Libraries Committee with an associated listserv. This group provides the opportunity to discuss accreditation with colleagues in similar situations who have gone through the process recently. It may also be helpful to look outside of librarianship for listservs and webinars. Medical schools or other health professions programs may have resources that they make available to individuals outside their institutions. After making connections via one of these strategies, pursuing a mentoring relationship with someone at another institution can provide the needed support to successfully navigate accreditation.

We live and work in a professional field, academic landscape, and world that is constantly growing and changing. Changes within our libraries and institutions add challenges to the already considerable challenge of accreditation. The addition of new health professions programs can bring with it fast-paced hiring and onboarding of new faces. This conclusion provides the key points to remember while navigating accreditation in times of growth and change, particularly for new libraries and programs.

It is impossible for a single person to be an expert in every library area that affects accreditation. Become familiar with the departments and people managing collections, electronic access, physical spaces, and health sciences services in order to ensure library resources and services are relevant and seamlessly accessible for the program. In the same vein, become as embedded in the medical school as is feasible, building relationships with key personnel and serving on relevant committees.

Personnel changes can add extra challenges to a successful accreditation cycle. Thorough and easily accessible documentation is the most important tool to successfully move through the process with a changing team.

Even clear documentation will not be enough if there is not also open, effective, and honest communication. Health sciences librarians need to be clear about how much support and what services they can realistically provide. It is important to be mindful of vocational awe and one's own capabilities and capacity. Setting expectations at the beginning of the process helps to build trust and leads to success.

Finally, accreditation is not the time to go it alone. Utilize the resources at your disposal, whatever shape they may take. Support can come from continuing education and professional organization resources, such as from MLA and AAHSL.

Colleagues within your institution may also have expertise on which to draw. Informal mentoring relationships are another valuable source of knowledge and support during accreditation.

While accreditation can feel especially challenging in times of accelerated growth and change, with appropriate preparation and planning, libraries and librarians can continue to successfully collaborate to contribute to the successful achievement of accreditation for health professions programs.

BIBLIOGRAPHY

Aslam, Mohammad. "Changing Behavior of Academic Libraries and the Role of Library Professionals," *Information Discovery and Delivery* 50, no. 1 (2021): 54–63, https://doi.org/10.1108/IDD-05-2020-0048.

Association of American Medical Colleges. "Approaches to the Independent Student Analysis: A Toolkit for Medical Students." Last modified September 2016. https://aamc-icollab.global.ssl.fastly.net/production/media/filer_public/36/a2/36a2c06a-18d5-49f7-8776-c787fae040c7/ic-resource-4336.pdf.

Liaison Committee on Medical Education. "Standards, Publications, & Notification Forms: LCME." Accessed January 15, 2022. https://lcme.org/publications/.

Thelin, John R., ed. *American Higher Education: Issues and Institutions.* New York and London: Routledge, 2017. https://ebookcentral.proquest.com/lib/uh/reader.action?docID=4809784&ppg=1.

University of Houston. "50-in-5." Last modified November 29, 2021. https://www.uh.edu/50-in-5/.

University of Houston. "Presidential Frontier Faculty." Office of the Provost. Last modified September 30, 2021. https://uh.edu/provost/faculty/prospective/pff/.

US Bureau of Labor Statistics. "Employee Tenure Summary." September 22, 2020. https://www.bls.gov/news.release/tenure.nr0.htm.

Wood, Barbara A., Ana B. Guimaraes, Christina E. Holm, Sherrill W. Hayes, and Kyle R. Brooks. "Academic Librarian Burnout: A Survey Using the Copenhagen Burnout Inventory (CBI)." *Journal of Library Administration* 60, no. 5 (2020): 5131, https://doi.org/10.1080/01930826.2020.1729622.

Wood, M. Sandra, ed. *Health Sciences Librarianship.* Lanham, MD: Rowman & Littlefield, 2014.

NOTES

1. M. Sandra Wood, *Health Sciences Librarianship* (Lanham, MD: Rowman & Littlefield, 2014), chap. 1, ProQuest Ebook Central.
2. John Thelin, *American Higher Education: Issues and Institutions* (New York and London: Routledge, 2017), chap. 2, Proquest Ebook Central.
3. "50-in-5," University of Houston, last modified November 29, 2021, https://www.uh.edu/50-in-5/.
4. "Presidential Frontiers Faculty," Office of the Provost, University of Houston, last modified September 30, 2021, https://uh.edu/provost/faculty/prospective/pff/.
5. Mohammad Aslam, "Changing Behavior of Academic Libraries and the Role of Library Professionals," *Information Discovery and Delivery* 50, no. 1 (2021): 7–8, https://doi.org/10.1108/IDD-05-2020-0048.
6. "Standards, Publications, & Notification Forms: LCME," Liaison Committee on Medical Education, accessed January 15, 2022, https://lcme.org/publications/.
7. "Approaches to the Independent Student Analysis: A Toolkit for Medical Students," Association of American Medical Colleges, last modified September 2016, https://aamc-icollab.global.ssl.fastly.net/production/media/filer_public/36/a2/36a2c06a-18d5-49f7-8776-c787fae040c7/ic-resource-4336.pdf, 5.
8. Wood, *Health Sciences Librarianship*, 210.
9. "Employee Tenure Summary," US Bureau of Labor Statistics, published September 22, 2020, https://www.bls.gov/news.release/tenure.nr0.htm.
10. Barbara A. Wood et al., "Academic Librarian Burnout: A Survey Using the Copenhagen Burnout Inventory (CBI)," *Journal of Library Administration* 60, no. 5 (2020): 512-31, https://doi.org/10.1080/01930826.2020.1729622.

4

First-Time Accreditation Process

LAYING THE GROUNDWORK

Connie Manning, Arkansas Colleges of Health Education; Sonya Lemke, Arkansas Colleges of Health Education; Darell Schmick, Noorda College of Osteopathic Medicine

When going through accreditation for the first time, there are a myriad of accompanying emotions—excitement and enthusiasm as well as anxiety and apprehension. The goal of this chapter is to provide an overview of what to expect throughout the process, with the caveat that there is much variability. Being prepared for any eventuality is key to positively navigating what can be a very changing and challenging landscape.

Most librarians experience first-time accreditations when their existing institutions are starting new programs, whereas the opportunity to create a library at a new institution is rare.[1] Today in the health sciences, both scenarios are occurring more frequently to address dire healthcare provider shortages.[2,3] This book is timely, filling in a literature gap on health sciences accreditation that was minimal until now. Yet another gap remains, that of creating libraries at new institutions and starting library services for new programs at existing institutions. The purpose of this chapter is to help with both gaps. As librarians who have recently gone through accreditation in both scenarios, the chapter authors share what they have learned about what to expect in laying the groundwork for first-time accreditation.

ASSESS THE SITUATION

A good initial step in the first-time accreditation process is to assess the situation, because not all firsts are the same. Is the institution a startup institution, or is it a new program at an existing institution? Which accreditations are the institution seeking, and what are the accrediting bodies? What are the differences between what the accreditation standards say and the institutional, mission-driven practices of the administrators, and do these differ from site visitors' perspectives? Each of these variables make going through accreditation for the first time unique.

NEW PROGRAMS AND NEW INSTITUTIONS

Starting from the ground up sounds very appealing—the chance to do it right the first time. However, unless experienced in starting a library at a new institution, it is easy to underestimate the amount of effort it takes or how fluid the process can be. Lofty goals for perfection quickly transition to doing your best, one day at a time. Again, very few librarians get this opportunity, so there is currently little guidance from the literature and professional organizations. Therefore, in the authors' experience, there are three characteristics of new institutions to consider.

One challenge at a new institution is the limited time and personnel in various departments. The library is no exception. It may take time to reach adequate staffing levels, and the staffing that is present is consumed with work. For example, the first library hire may be the only intended library personnel (whether the title is simply medical/health sciences librarian, library director, or library dean) with no immediate plans for growth in staffing. If that is the intention, either initially or even for a few years, preparing for accreditation is another responsibility that demands attention in a very hefty to-do list. Yet, even if you are the solo librarian building a library from scratch and preparing for potentially multiple initial accreditations, know that you are not alone. The health sciences librarian community is active through professional organizations, such as the Medical Library Association (MLA) and the Association of Academic Health Sciences Libraries (AAHSL). A good use of your limited time in the beginning is connecting to this community, so consider prioritizing travel to conferences your first couple of years. Attendance offers visibility for you and your institution and provides great networking opportunities with the chance to make lasting connections with colleagues in the field. You might even connect with someone who is in a situation like yours. If travel is not an option, another avenue for help is to consider bringing in a consultant. However, like attending professional meetings, this is dependent on having a budget for these activities. If it is possible, having another voice advocating for the library, and specifically one from outside the institution, can add additional support to your plans for building the library and provide you with needed guidance.

Another distinguishing feature of new institutions is the abundance of new perspectives. A new institution has employees who are new to the professional workforce, those who are mid-career, and those nearing retirement. There are employees who are not new to health sciences and clinical practice but are new to academic health sciences or their current role and responsibilities in academia. Finally, there are employees who are new to the specific fields of health sciences that the institution offers, such as moving to an osteopathic medical school after previously working at a medical school. With this diversity of perspectives and experiences at startups, it is common to hear during the creation of policies, procedures, and plans, "Well, at my former institution, we did it this way." While that statement can be viewed negatively if the speaker isn't willing to consider new ideas or listen to other's perspectives, there is also a positive aspect in hearing this repetitive statement. All the employees of a new institution bring a spectrum of perspectives and experiences that, when paired with evidence and best practices, provides breadth and value in the creation process.

This panoply of ideas at new institutions is part of the excitement of startups, but it is also a symptom of an unfortunately common occurrence—turnover. Academic medicine turnover is a known issue. In a 2018 paper, Nausheen cites American Association of Medical Colleges (AAMC) data confirming "that 38% of faculty overall and 43% of first-time assistant professors leave academic medicine within a 10-year period, and that first-time assistant professors with both MD and PhD degrees were more likely to switch medical schools."[4] Documentation for even greater turnover at new institutions is sparse, as Nausheen notes, but all three authors can anecdotally attest to this.[5] At new institutions, the sheer number and frequency of changes take a toll on the most experienced academicians and clinicians. Just as there is a spectrum of employees and their experiences, a spectrum also applies toward their attitudes in working at a new institution. Some, attracted to startups for the animated atmosphere, stay for a few years and then leave for another startup, ready for another challenge. Others, attracted by the opportunities but overwhelmed by the rigorous setting, may experience burnout and choose to leave. Those who stay long term acknowledge the effort and perseverance it takes managing the stresses of a new institution, usually because they are passionate about the institution's impact and the mission of the institution.

What do these three observations of new institutions mean for the library? Turnover (and its accompanying new perspectives) in key roles relating to the library administration can affect the library's progress. While personnel changes are welcome if there is a better alignment of vision for the library or if opportunities open that were previously closed, changes will be mixed. For example, when a change in committee chair occurred, one of the authors was able to finally get on a research committee, which often is valuable for the library. For another author, an experience of turnover was neither positive nor negative; it was problematic due to frequency. The administrator to whom the head of the library reports changed five times in as many years. With each new hire bringing a different set of experiences and ideas about the role of the library, it took time adjusting and aligning their perspectives with the library director's each time there was a change. Changes in other departments can affect the library as well if the departments work intimately with aspects of library work, such as academic affairs, finance, or information technology. How to weather such changes without losing too much momentum is discussed more in depth in the section below on planning.

In addition to the effects of limited time and limited personnel discussed above, another situation regarding staffing is that a sizable portion of library planning may have occurred before the first library hire is even made. Institutional administrators may have the library space, resources budget, and staffing requirements determined with little to no collaboration with library personnel.[6] In her article "Library Startup: Reflections on Building a New Community College Library from Scratch," Reed describes her efforts to build the library, but it is not truly from scratch, as much was already in place.[7] Before her hire, there was a predecessor and additional staff member, a library website and integrated library system, and a designated library space with "roughly 3,000 monographs" that were "the library's first and most substantial book purchase."[8] For one of the authors of this chapter, no books had been purchased before the first library hire, but the library space was already designated (with office space for only one librarian). The space was furnished with study carrels, bookshelves, even a book cart—although the vision for the library was to have almost a completely digital library. On the flip side, if the first library hire does have the opportunity to completely design the library's digital and physical spaces and resources in collaboration with administrators, seize that opportunity. Here is the chance to take the perspectives and experiences of all involved and pair them with evidence and best practices. Consider using usability studies from institutions like yours in your planning, which may strengthen discussions with an accreditor.

NEW PROGRAMS AT EXISTING INSTITUTIONS

The other scenario for experiencing first-time accreditation is when new programs join existing institutions. For example, suppose an existing college or university opts to build a medical school or add multiple allied health programs. There is a formidable amount of established structure to navigate for new programs, in addition to the employees hired for this purpose. Though there are no clear advantages or disadvantages between the two scenarios, there are things to keep in mind when you are part of a team bringing a new program to an existing institution.

First, familiarize yourself with the existing culture and infrastructure. It is important to note that the parent institution has a vision and a mission already in place. The new program should fit into this greater mission rather than exist independently. It would serve the new program well to align goals to be complementary to this institution. This is especially true for the library. Consider what library groundwork exists. Does the existing institution already have a library in place? Does the program have a library team hired to support it, or is it an accountability of an existing subject librarian? The library's reporting obligation is important to note as well. If the program operates with greater autonomy, the library may report to an associate dean or dean. If the program is established within a greater college or school, the library may be responsible to the university library.

In both configurations, it is to the program's benefit that it have an advocate for its library needs. A new health sciences program may have anywhere from moderate to significant requirements tethered to the availability of library resources that programmatic leadership requires. In the case of existing programs, a university may have resources already within the area of health sciences. Therefore, a comprehensive audit of available resources and the program's needs should be conducted. Ensuring the library has a point of contact in the program's curriculum, as well as a voice on the collection development committee (if the library has one), would serve to keep communication clear on this need. If sharing a budget with the greater university, be sure to articulate the importance of obtaining certain resources while being sensitive to other disciplines' needs. A health sciences program may cost more to fund through full accreditation than a humanities program, but it is important to know that each of these disciplines has a place in the greater campus community.

An institution undergoing growth may have stories and tensions that precede employees that are just joining. New employees hired to help with the program's inception may not fully appreciate the history leading up to the program's launch. The decision to bring on the program could have been an unpopular one. Or it could have been a popular one, but with several unpopular decisions executed in the meantime. Each of these situations has the potential of adding to the stress of the collective campus. It is important to be reminded that there may not be a perfect rollout. Newcomers and veterans alike should take comfort in knowing that the decisions of today supplant the decisions made in the past. There is no sense in dwelling when there is much work to be done.

Some of the most valuable colleagues during the excitement of starting a new program will be those who have institutional knowledge. While newcomers to the institution will be acculturated to processes and procedures, they still can come up short next to a veteran who has submitted multiple budgets from years past at the institution or the person who is familiar with the most easily accessible point persons within a given department. These colleagues, whether they have transferred to a role within the program or work alongside it, are indispensable assets with their wisdom.

ACCREDITATION BASICS

Equipped with the knowledge of what to expect with new programs at new institutions and existing institutions, the next step is to learn the basics of accreditation. Outside of leadership positions, most librarians generally encounter the accreditation process as part of their liaison responsibilities. You may have been asked to prepare in full or supply information for an accreditation report. You may even have participated in the site visit. If now you are assuming responsibility for accreditations already in process or pursuing first-time accreditation, a foundational understanding of how accreditation works is necessary.

As discussed more in depth in chapter 1, there are two types of accreditations that an academic institution works toward: institutional and programmatic. For first-time accreditations, a few special circumstances are of note. First, programmatic accreditors require an institution to have institutional accreditation. Of those, some accreditors may require an institution to obtain full accreditation before it can apply for its programmatic accreditation. Others will accept an application if the institution has at least candidacy status. There are some programmatic accreditors, such as the Commission on Osteopathic College Accreditation (COCA), that can serve as both the institutional and programmatic accreditor when it is the only program of an institution, in this case a free-standing college of osteopathic medicine. Second, accrediting bodies may offer different routes to achieving accreditation. For example, the Higher Learning Commission, one of the six regional institutional accreditors, offers (1) eligibility process and candidacy, and (2) accelerated process for initial accreditation. A new institution may be ambitious to pursue multiple accreditations simultaneously or closely staggered, with some via the accelerated routes. In the next stage of laying the groundwork, planning, it is important to discuss an accreditation timeline with all accreditations laid out, but being cognizant that plans, even for onboarding programs, can change.

STANDARDS VERSUS PRACTICES

ACCREDITATION STANDARDS

Now that you are familiar with what to expect regarding your institutional situation and the accreditation process, take time to look at the standards in detail. Remember how you have administrators and colleagues with a diversity of perspectives and experiences? Many will have input regarding how to achieve the standards regarding the library. Listen to them, but also carefully review the standards yourself. Some of what you are told may be a case of "Well, at my former institution, we did it this way." However, there are three objective reasons why you should go to the source.

First, with a good number of health sciences accrediting bodies, it is not surprising that the standards of each vary regarding the library. And some standards may not mention a library at all. Instead, you may see references to required "learning resources" that are clumped together with student services, simulation, and question banks. If applying to multiple accrediting bodies, take note of where there are differences and overlaps; this information is valuable in the planning process. Second, accrediting bodies can have different standards for the different stages of the accreditation process. Using COCA again as an example, there are two sets of standards: (1) those for "new and developing" programs, and (2) those for "continuing programs." Consider the different sets and see if there are differences regarding the library between the two.

Last, be aware that the standards of accreditation bodies change over time. Divergent input you receive from an administrator or library colleague may not be based on practices at their former institution, but instead on former standards. If seeking or receiving help, be sure to know when their institution last went through accreditation. Changes can even occur during the middle of your institution's planning. These changes can be minor or major. They can also be looser or stricter. Also, it is not unheard of for an institution to start under one set of standards and then change to new standards midway through, since the process of accreditation takes time. A program may have to adjust its onboarding timeline if eligibility requirements change, creating a trickle-down effect in the institution. If the library was planning to onboard resources at a certain start date, those resources may be postponed and thus the budget adjusted for the new timeline.

CURRENT (AND FORMER) INSTITUTIONAL PRACTICES

Accreditation standards generally do not list or define specific requirements, but that does not mean that an administrator's perspective or practice in achieving a set of standards is not valuable. Remember that an institution's mission will impact institutional practices. If a practice is based on standards that have changed, are from another field, or are the practices of a former institution, now is a good chance to align the administrator's input with your vision of what is best, as well as what evidence and best practices say. For example, one of the authors was told by an administrator that the library needed three copies of each required textbook. Yet the standards for that program do not specify how many textbooks are required in print. Instead, for a primarily digital library, this practice could be considered useful in case of digital access issues or as a stopgap for students waiting to purchase books until financial aid is released.

Another author example is when a new program's dean requested the library have a copy of an important textbook for each student. Fifty copies of only one textbook would be impractical to purchase due to the library's obligations to all constituencies. It would also be impractical to have copies on the stacks in the event the textbooks were not purchased from the library's budget. An existing, well-written, and public-facing collection development policy can shield the library from such predicaments. A collection development policy that provides a maximum number of books of one specific edition would demonstrate the library has a limit to which considered books will be purchased. You could even consider defining which sort of textbooks the library will purchase, if any, to ensure a greater diversity of a collection that supports the curriculum.

New programs provide the opportunity for those involved to develop a greater understanding as to what libraries can do for them. Decision makers may have varying degrees of understanding of libraries, and even our most well-versed and supportive administrators or department heads outside of the library may be operating on outdated norms. Therefore, transparency in library operating procedures is valuable to have at the outset. Providing library operations procedures to administrators, particularly collection development policies, donation policies, and policies regarding space usage, can demonstrate objectivity in how the library (and the corresponding collection) is managed. Publishing these policies on the library website allows for library patrons (administrators included) to view these before making requests that fall outside of the parameters of the library's responsibilities.

PLAN, AND PLAN TO BE FLEXIBLE

With the situation assessed and foundational knowledge acquired, it is time to plan. The amount of planning and the strengths of those plans are going to be contingent on factors in and outside of your control. Since you are seeking accreditation the first time, it is natural to strive for perfection, doing all things right the first time. But that is an unrealistic goal. Instead, do the best planning you can. Take suggestions from this section and make them your own. And take to heart this quote from thirty-fourth US President Dwight D. Eisenhower: "Plans are worthless, but planning is everything."[9] Especially in first-time accreditation, the process of planning itself is more important because plans will change.

SETTING UP A COMMUNICATIONS PLAN FOR THE LIBRARY

It is a good idea to have a communication strategy for the library, preferably in writing. For something as significant as accreditation, knowing what to communicate to which constituency and when can minimize confusion. With first-time accreditations occurring as a kaleidoscope of scenarios, start by simply establishing who is going to communicate with whom. As mentioned earlier, the planning of a new institution or a new program may often involve library planning prior to the hiring of any library personnel. However, once onboarded it is imperative that relevant library personnel meet with leadership to understand what their vision and expectations are of the library. Having a meeting early allows all parties to map out a plan for success in the years to follow. You may be the point person or part of the team that will be ensuring a communications plan is in place. The library director is the logical point person as the library representative in most organizational structures, but liaison librarians and the university librarian may be involved as well.

If you are a solo librarian at a new institution, you will have a communication channel established with your immediate supervisor regarding the institution's expectations of the library. But how will you connect with programmatic leadership? And how will you make sure that institutional and programmatic expectations regarding the library align? Will you meet one-on-one with each program leader, or all together with your immediate supervisor? If you are solo at first but then you hire additional library personnel, will communications with programmatic leadership become part of their roles, say, as part of a liaison model, with you involved to varying extent? If not, you will still need to keep them and your entire team in the loop to ensure they are kept informed. As for librarians leading new programs at existing institutions, consider these questions: What is the library's relationship with the university library? Is there independence in communicating with the program leadership or are communications required to go through the university librarian? How are supporting library staff kept informed? For example, you may have mostly liaison librarians at your library, whereas the librarians that handle technical services and systems work solely at the university library.

For all these scenarios, consider all perspectives of those who interact with the library when drafting a strategy—who needs to be informed, what they need to know, and when. Each reporting relationship has a variety of means in which you communicate. Know which ones are most effective and prepare accordingly. For instance, your immediate supervisor may have a significant role in compiling the report for the site visit and may prefer to communicate via email. Your direct reports within the library may prefer to receive information at library staff or leadership meetings. Library patrons may be most effectively informed by posting pertinent information on the library website. Knowing the most effective communication method for each constituency is valuable in a successful strategy. Finally, plan for the constituency in mind. The information will be most beneficial targeted to the role and audience as opposed to the person(s) in those roles, especially if there is turnover. Knowing what to prioritize when communicating with leadership will allow for more impactful interactions; they are pressed for time as accreditation timelines get closer. It will also allow for the leadership team to temper expectations accordingly.

Your communications strategy will likely have successes as well as future opportunities. In establishing communication channels, you may not be successful for every program. For example, you may believe that you should be on a certain council or committee that would provide institutional or programmatic feedback, such as provost's council or a program curriculum committee. If your immediate supervisor says no, you must work with what you have. And because of that, there will be times when planning misses the mark. An example is reactively having to acquire an expensive resource that was not communicated to you and thus not budgeted. In such circumstances, diplomatically point out these are reasons that you need to be on said council or committee. Take this opportunity to ask questions about future planning and the participation of the library.

NEEDS, WANTS, AND EXPECTATIONS

With communications channels established, evaluate the needs, wants, and expectations of all parties involved. If working on multiple accreditations, consider creating a crosswalk of all accreditation standards regarding the library. This is a good idea even if you are not facing accreditation for the first time. The needs and wants of one program may overlap with another.

Before going over the specifics of this resource versus that, ask the program leadership which metrics they consider necessary for the program's success. Determine what the library currently has in place to meet those metrics. If they do not have metrics in mind, ask the program leadership if they are modeling a program at another institution. If they are, ask for what was used to create and measure their outcomes. The program dean's office will almost certainly have these. Keep in mind, a program is not required to provide a template of their metrics. They can do so if they choose. If you are looking online, be sure to verify you are referring to the latest iteration of the templates and trust only official sources, such as the accrediting body main webpage. If there is such a program, getting an idea as to available resources at that institution's library (as well as a point of contact for librarians who have gone down this path before) is an excellent resource. If there isn't a program the leadership is modeling, look for established programs that are similar in mission to yours, or look to similar new programs coming on. For example, in 2017 an informal group of new library directors at osteopathic schools formed FOLD (Founding Osteopathic Library Directors) because there were multiple new osteopathic schools starting around the same time.[10] Reaching out and building communities of colleagues is one of the best resources utilized in the first-time accreditation process.

After learning what metrics and what program models the leadership has in mind, it is time to set realistic expectations with the programs and the institution. Recall that you may have administrators who are new to certain health sciences fields, academia, or their role. Additionally, they may have little or outdated experience with libraries and the acquisitions of library resources. For example, at one of the author's institutions, the initial budget for the library—planned before the first library hire—was drastically inadequate. By quickly reviewing what resources were at similar institutions and contacting vendors for quotes, the librarian was able to provide documentation that aligned the institution's initial expectations with a realistic resources budget.

Aligning expectations also requires being aware of both institutional and programmatic accreditation timelines. For best success, request the program timelines from leadership. What will it take and how long will it take for this program to be fully accredited? Consider embedding regular check-ins as a team throughout the process. Besides discussing resources and services, clarify with leadership what they need for documentation, and when. You will want to budget as far in advance as you can, but plan for flexibility, because changes can and probably will happen. If your administration is firm on a more limited initial budget, accept less-than-perfect resources and systems with the knowledge that you can later scale up. An institution and its programs grow over time; so will the library.

LIBRARY PRACTICES THAT SUPPORT DOCUMENTATION

With so many changes and so much out of your control, you can take strength in keeping the library functioning and effective throughout the accreditation process. Below are three strategies that you can use to plan. First, keep all accreditation reports and documentation in one location. Decide who will be responsible for maintaining the reports and documents, as well as the location. Documentation is generally submitted electronically. Therefore, consider adopting a file-naming convention. Descriptive file names are important to organize, share, and keep track of the files. Having organized files makes finding the correct requested document fast and efficient. Check with the point of contact at your institution assigned to collect and send documentation whether the institution or the accrediting body uses a file-naming convention. If not, create your own. For example, CAPTE_Library_Narrative_2021.06.15_toAnderson.pdf describes that the file is for the Commission on Accreditation in Physical Therapy Education (CAPTE) accreditation, the library portion, the deliverable type, the date (in YYYY.DD.MM for sorting) and the recipient's last name. This may seem excessive but remember that institutional turnover is never out of the question and the current person may not have access to the deliverable that you turned in to their predecessor. Keeping all documentation, regardless of it becoming obsolete for future accreditation cycles, is valuable historical data that tells the story of the library's growth.

Second, consider adding metadata to records, such as MARC records, that identify which program or programs the resources support. Some libraries may utilize separate budget lines as well. Quality metadata about programs helps with quickly supplying information for accreditation reports, but also for other reports such as statistics reporting. Finally, look for efficiencies in reporting. Recall that accrediting standards are not specific generally. There are no glossaries of library-focused definitions the way there are for reporting to the Integrated Postsecondary Education Data System (IPEDS). Pull out the crosswalk, if you made one, for your multiple programs and ask whether they all exhibit a level of flexibility in the reporting requirements. If so, consider using the more rigorous reporting guidelines of other administrative reports, such as IPEDS, so that you are not duplicating efforts. For example, in reporting library resources, should open-access resources be included? Should resources be specific only to the program, to the health sciences, or to the entire campus, which may include fields outside of the health sciences? If you are not using the standards of IPEDS or AAHSL as your baseline, make sure you document the decision process for how you reported data for the accreditation report.

STAND AND DELIVER

At this point, a theme is clearly visible—successfully navigating accreditation requires flexibility owing to the amount of variability. The final push is no different. As described below, deliverables, such as reports and tables, differ not only in style but in content as well, depending on the standards of the accrediting body. Site visits that are customary regarding with whom site visitors meet and the questions they ask are less so with respect to the library. Be prepared that after all the work involved, the library may not be listed on the visit agenda. Instead, you may be on call in case the accreditors have a question. Plan for all scenarios.

DELIVERABLES

The accreditation process is never truly complete. Expect to produce accreditation deliverables for your administration on a regular basis as planned. That said, while deliverables, such as reports and tables, are anticipated at certain stages of the process for the initial and continuing accreditation, keep in mind that deliverables can be requested at any time as part of an audit. The type of deliverable itself usually does not change from the initial stage to the continuing stage (unless the standards themselves change), but the content of the deliverable should change as you continue to build the library's collection. Having planned to keep clearly identified files for each instance of a deliverable's submission is beneficial, again, not just for good record keeping and a means of tracking programs' collection growth but also for any spur-of-the-moment request from administration.

The most common deliverable that is requested of the library is a narrative or report, whereas the most compact deliverable the authors have encountered is a solitary table. Narratives require a response consisting of descriptive evidence that supports the narrative's request. For example, the CAPTE standards require the following: "Describe the adequacy of the library resources, including the technological resources, and related learning resource centers available to the program faculty and students."[11] To provide evidence for this broad request, the library must decide how much evidence is adequate. There are some consistent pieces of information that libraries usually report: number of personnel and their qualifications, physical size of the library space and furnishing information, total number of resources, list of services, and so on. Some accreditors will require additional information such as the entire library budget or just the portion dedicated to the program in question, physical and digital accessibility parameters, and more detailed information on resources (licensing concurrency, subscription versus all access, including open access).

SITE VISITS

After months (maybe a couple of years) of planning, and after weeks or months since turning in deliverables, it is finally time for the site visit—or more accurately, site visits. Yes, there can be more than one. A site visit is the institution's opportunity to showcase not only the facilities but, more importantly, all the enthusiastic and well-informed personnel who have worked hard building the programs and preparing all those accreditation deliverables. Being nervous at the first site visit in your first accreditation is understandable, but remember that you are the expert regarding the library. No one knows that content better than you. Just keep in mind that for the site visit and, as you've seen, for the entire process, being flexible will ensure the library has a successful visit.

To help the institution prepare for these important visits, some institutions conduct mock visits. Mock visits provide the opportunity to simulate closely the process of the actual visit. Consultants with experience in accreditations and site visits may be brought in to lead a mock visit. Not only are these visits a good means to practice and work through any nerves, but they can also be a way to share knowledge about the library with others in your institution whose interactions with the library up to this point may have been peripheral. Take advantage of all mock visits to promote the library and to practice, but do so respectfully and strategically.

Just as the library's role varies among accreditation standards, so does the library's role in site visits. If an accrediting body has minimal language regarding the library in its standards, expect the library's role in the site visit to be minimal as well. In fact, the library may not even be on the schedule but is instructed to be available upon request. If the library is on the schedule, it may be included with other departments. In the case of a shared session, be prepared to know important information regarding the institution, such as the mission of the institution or the program. Likewise, you will be responsible for that information and more if you serve on committees also on the schedule, such as curriculum, grants, or research. If fortunate to have a site visit session devoted solely to the library, take the opportunity to boast about the library. However, be succinct and adjust your responses depending on whether the site visitor you meet with is a librarian, as described in more detail in chapter 7.

Finally, as the authors are writing this chapter in 2022, it is worth noting that even the most flexible and accustomed can be surprised. Site visits, as the terminology implies, occur "on site" but pandemics, as well as natural disasters, obligate change. Just as many in the world have become closely familiar with video teleconferencing technologies, so have academic institutions and accrediting bodies. Site visit meetings scheduled to occur in physical rooms were shifted to meetings in virtual rooms. Walking tours of the campus were transformed into prerecorded, high-production video tours. Going forward, site visits may incorporate these new methods of connecting with the institution being evaluated as a matter of course and not just in extenuating circumstances.

CONCLUSION

Undertaking a significant endeavor for the first time can be challenging. There will be things that could have been done differently. There will be things that were out of one's control and unforeseen. What is important in going through a first is that you did it. You persevered, you learned from it, and hopefully you shared what you learned with others. Starting library services at a new institution is a monumental task and hard work. And starting new programs, especially multiple programs concurrently, is no simple feat. Going through accreditation is one piece of this first. The authors hope that in sharing their insights and reflections on their first-time accreditations, those who get this opportunity will have a clearer understanding of the process and be prepared for whatever their first entails.

NOTES

1. Kim Leeder Reed, "Library Startup: Reflections on Building a New Community College Library from Scratch," *Journal of Library Administration* 56, no. 5 (2016): 621–27, https://doi.org/10.1080/01930826.2016.1186971.

2. Nadine Dexter et al., "Building New Twenty-First Century Medical School Libraries from the Ground Up: Challenges, Experiences, and Lessons Learned," *Journal of the Medical Library Association* 107, no. 1 (2019): 6–15, https://doi.org/doi:10.5195/jmla.2019.493.

3. Fauzia Nausheen et al., "A Survey of Retaining Faculty at a New Medical School: Opportunities, Challenges and Solutions," *BMC Medical Education* 18, no. 1 (2018), https://doi.org/10.1186/s12909-018-1330-z.

4. Nausheen, "Survey," 2.

5. Nausheen, "Survey," abstract.

6. Nancy Fried Foster, "Designing a New Academic Library from Scratch," *Ithaka S+R* (2014). https://doi.org/10.18665/sr.24776.

7. Reed, "Library Startup."

8. Reed, "Library Startup," 623.

9. Dwight D. Eisenhower, "Speech to the National Defense Executive Reserve Conference in Washington, D.C., November 14, 1957," in *Public Papers of the Presidents of the United States, Dwight D. Eisenhower, 1957*, edited by Government Printing Office, National Archives and Records Service.

10. Darell Schmick et al., "Bringing Each Other into the FOLD: Shared Experiences in Start-Up Osteopathic Medical School Libraries" (poster, Annual Conference of the Medical Library Association, Atlanta, GA, May 22, 2018). https://doi.org/10.5195/jmla.2019.672.

11. Commission on Accreditation in Physical Therapy Education, *Standards and Required Elements for Accreditation of Physical Therapist Education Programs* (Alexandria, VA: American Physical Therapy Association, 2021).

BIBLIOGRAPHY

Commission on Accreditation in Physical Therapy Education. *Standards and Required Elements for Accreditation of Physical Therapist Education Programs*. Alexandria, VA: American Physical Therapy Association, 2021.

Dexter, Nadine, Joanne M. Muellenbach, Elizabeth R. Lorbeer, Debra Rand, Matthew E. Wilcox, and Bradley A. Long. "Building New Twenty-First Century Medical School Libraries from the Ground Up: Challenges, Experiences, and Lessons Learned." *Journal of the Medical Library Association* 107, no. 1 (2019): 6–15. https://doi.org/doi:10.5195/jmla.2019.493.

Eisenhower, Dwight D. "Speech to the National Defense Executive Reserve Conference in Washington, D.C., November 14, 1957." In *Public Papers of the Presidents of the United States, Dwight D. Eisenhower, 1957*, edited by Government Printing Office, National Archives and Records Service.

Foster, Nancy F. "Designing a New Academic Library from Scratch." *Ithaka S+R* (2014). https://doi.org/doi.org/10.18665/sr.24776.

Nausheen, Fauzia, Mukesh M. Agarwal, John J. Estrada, and Dhammika N. Atapattu. "A Survey of Retaining Faculty at a New Medical School: Opportunities, Challenges and Solutions." *BMC Medical Education* 18, no. 1 (2018). https://doi.org/10.1186/s12909-018-1330-z.

Reed, Kim L. "Library Startup: Reflections on Building a New Community College Library from Scratch." *Journal of Library Administration* 56, no. 5 (2016): 621–27. https://doi.org/10.1080/01930826.2016.1186971.

Schmick, Darell, Elizabeth Wright, Erin Palazzolo, Norice Lee, Molly Montgomery, and Anna Yang. "Bringing Each Other into the FOLD: Shared Experiences in Start-Up Osteopathic Medical School Libraries." Poster presented at the Annual Conference of the Medical Library Association, Atlanta, GA, May 22, 2018. https://doi.org/10.5195/jmla.2019.672.

Part Two

The Accreditation Process

5

Ongoing Accreditation Efforts

MAGNET RECOGNITION AND THE ROLE OF THE LIBRARIAN

Roy Brown and Alison Montpetit, Virginia Commonwealth University

Healthcare in the United States is evolving and ever more complex because of increasing demands on the system. These demands are a result of several factors. First is the increasing acuity and morbidity of patients. Second, patients have more options for care and utilize the increased accessibility of information to inform their choices on where to receive care. Third, healthcare providers must address issues regarding expanding access to health insurance and healthcare brought on by government policies. These challenges must be met while also managing the challenges of changing workforce trends, cost containment, pay-for-performance incentives, and reimbursement constraints. The healthcare environment is made more complex as healthcare organizations must also meet key performance indicators that address patient satisfaction, thirty-day readmission rates, and other measures related to patient safety. These cost-containment demands are further pushed by private payers and insurance companies that require evidence-based interventions. As a result, healthcare providers participate in interdisciplinary, patient-centered care where current care standards are evaluated, and new solutions are created based on the most up-to-date evidence. Nurses constitute the largest healthcare provider workforce, with 2.9 million registered nurses employed in the United States, compared with 713,800 physicians and surgeons.[1]

When it comes to healthcare, nurses provide holistic care that spans the continuum of care from ambulatory to acute care to the community and the systems level. This approach to patient care differs from other healthcare disciplines that tend to be more disease, procedure, or specialty focused. As a result of their broad participation, nurses are well positioned to make impactful changes but only if empowered to question practice and implement solutions. The 2004 Institute of Medicine report titled *Keeping Patients Safe: Transforming the Work Environment of Nurses* recognizes this ability to impact patient safety positively. This report identified organizational structures that are accentuated by strong nursing leadership and adequate nurse staffing which are crucial to providing safe patient care. Unfortunately, like many other disciplines in the pressured healthcare system, the nursing workforce faces stressful work environments, exposure to violence in the healthcare setting, and challenges with staffing ratios. These issues lead to burnout, compassion fatigue, turnover, and retention issues.

In addition, the loss of experienced nurses at the bedside places additional pressure on an already stressed healthcare system.[2] Many nursing organizations, including the American Nurses Association (ANA), have recognized these factors. The ANA recognizes that nurses make up the largest workforce in a hospital, constituting 40 percent of operating costs while at the same time facing cutbacks like reduced hours and staffing.[3] This leads to threats to patient safety and nurse welfare. Because of these issues, the American Academy of Nursing in 1981

14 Forces of Magnetism	
1.	Quality of Nursing Leadership
2.	Organizational Structure
3.	Management Style
4.	Personnel Policies and Programs
5.	Professional Models of Care
6.	Quality of Care
7.	Quality Improvement
8.	Consultation and Resources
9.	Autonomy
10.	Community and the Hospital
11.	Nurses as Teachers
12.	Image of Nursing
13.	Interdisciplinary Relationships
14.	Professional Development

Figure 5.1. 14 Forces of Magnetism
SOURCE: ROY BROWN

commissioned a study to investigate the factors that impeded or facilitated professional nursing practice in hospitals. The four researchers who conducted the study understood that healthcare faced a nursing shortage. However, some hospitals succeeded in attracting and retaining well-qualified nurses and consistently providing quality care.[4] As a result of the study, fourteen nursing professional practice environment characteristics were identified. These were called the Forces of Magnetism.[5] These forces help develop a culture that supports nursing practice and quality patient care (see figure 5.1).

The fourteen Forces of Magnetism were the foundation of the American Nurses Association's framework in 1990 to develop a program to evaluate organizational nursing excellence, which was overseen by the American Nurses Credentialing Center (ANCC). The program developed was the Magnet Recognition Program. The standards that a Magnet organization is judged upon are no longer the fourteen Forces of Magnetism. In 2020, the standards were distilled down to the five Magnet Model Components. The components still incorporate the original fourteen forces to provide a clearer nursing practice and research framework. The transition also hopes to streamline documentation for meeting the goals and help place a greater focus on outcomes.[6] These six new components are:

- **Organizational Overview (OO):** Describes various aspects of the organization.
- **Empirical Outcomes (EO):** Measures nursing's contribution to measurable outcomes in patient care, nursing work environment, and others.
- **Transformational Leadership (TL):** Empowers leadership to ensure nurses at all levels have a voice that is heard, valued, incorporated in decision making, and practice supported to transform care and the work environment.
- **Structural Empowerment (SE):** Involves clinical nurses in shared governance, decision making, and establishing standards of practice.
- **Exemplary Professional Practice (EP):** The existence of a robust Professional Practice Model and how it defines, shapes, and influences care and positive patient and workforce outcomes.
- **New Knowledge, Innovations & Improvements (NK):** Nursing Inquiry and Innovation, including the translation of evidence into practice, performance improvement, innovations, and the generation of new knowledge through research.

The Magnet Commission frames these domains within Standards of Excellence (SOEs) that are revised every four years to reflect the most current trends within the profession. Currently, there are more than one hundred SOEs, with over twenty of those focusing on research, evidence-based practice, or performance improvement.[7] Through the evaluation process to receive Magnet recognition, hospitals and healthcare organizations are recognized for providing nurses with a culture of empowerment that leads to improved patient outcomes to recruit high-quality nurses and demonstrate the ability to retain them. Presently there are 547 Magnet-designated organizations worldwide.[8]

LIBRARIAN SUPPORT OF MAGNET RECOGNITION

Virginia Commonwealth University (VCU) Health is an 811-bed, urban academic medical, level 1 trauma center in Richmond, Virginia. The organization is composed of more than 3,500 nurses and more than 40 PhD- or DNP-prepared nurses. It is a four-time Magnet accredited institution with thirteen designated American Association of Critical Care Nurses Beacon Units. Each of these is an organizational and unit-level recognition of excellence, respectively. In addition, the hospital has strong academic partnerships with both the VCU School of Nursing and the VCU Libraries Health Sciences Library.

The Health Science Library (HSL) is a part of VCU Libraries, including the James Branch Cabell Library, a general academic library. Since 1994 the HSL has had a school-based liaison program focused on providing services to the faculty, staff, and students to meet their research, clinical, and educational needs. Each school and discipline has an assigned medical librarian as a liaison. The health sciences campus of VCU is comprised of five schools: medicine, nursing, pharmacy, dentistry, and health professions, with a combined enrollment of more than five thousand students who attend face-to-face, online, and hybrid programs. This campus also serves the VCU Medical Center, the Children's Hospital of Richmond at VCU, and a satellite campus at Community Memorial Hospital located in South Hill, Virginia.

The medical librarian in this framework serves the members of the VCU School of Nursing and the nurses of VCU Health. In this role, starting in 2010, the medical librarian for nursing began supporting the organization and became more deeply involved with VCU Health nursing in 2015 as the organization prepared for its third Magnet redesignation. The designation or redesignation process presents an opportunity to reflect on organizational processes and outcomes. During this time, the organization recognized the role of the library, specifically the role the medical librarian could play in supporting Magnet recognition.

At VCU, the library's main impact has been supporting the Standards of Excellence (SOE) that are a part of the New Knowledge, Innovations, and Improvements (NK) component of the Magnet Model Components. Essential to this component, the library is responsible for maintaining a collection that contains new evidence publications that are key in developing new standards of care or translating research findings to the bedside. Clinical inquiry is key to the NK component, and nurses need to be able to engage meaningfully in the evidence-based practice (EBP) process. EBP requires that nurses know how to question current practice, access evidence, and apply it within the practice environment. A nurse's past clinical experience and current patient needs also play a role in the process. Using evidence to guide practice ensures that patients receive the best care regardless of where they receive it and offers a strategy for reducing clinical variation across an organization. In the healthcare environment, evidence can empower nurses to engage meaningfully in an interdisciplinary approach and lead the team to evaluate current practice and translate new knowledge to improve patient care while containing costs.

According to the Institute of Medicine report *Crossing the Quality Chasm* and other studies, it currently takes an average of seventeen years for new knowledge generated by research to be translated and incorporated into practice.[9,10,11] The seventeen-year delay in incorporating new knowledge into practice is problematic. This delay in translating evidence is especially concerning because the National Academies of Sciences, Engineering, and Medicine, in a 2008 report, stated that the goal for healthcare was to have 90 percent of all healthcare decisions be evidence-based by 2020.[12] Presently, healthcare is lagging in utilizing evidence with only about 18 percent of the recommendations based on high-quality evidence. In contrast, nearly half are based on expert opinion, usual care, or disease-oriented evidence.[13] One reason for the lack of an evidence base for a significant portion of nursing practice is that nursing has been traditionally viewed as a service profession compared to other healthcare disciplines like medicine. Nursing has a relatively young science base when it comes to nursing practice, and as a result, the skill development in EBP is still ongoing. This has led to skill development in EBP not being valued or viewed as a priority in nursing practice; it is not fully understood as to what it means to be competent when it comes to EBPs.

Additionally, this is further impacted by the various levels of education (diploma, associate, baccalaureate degree) pipelines into the nursing profession. Some of these programs do not offer EBP and research preparation; therefore, some nurses entering the workforce may lack the skills to effectively engage in the EBP research process.[14,15,16,17] The EBP skill deficit is not from a lack of interest. Even when interested in EBP, nurses report facing barriers like lack of time, knowledge of the process, mentorship, and organizational support.[18,19,20] Part of this may be because executive leadership has not yet recognized the value and importance of nursing involvement with EBP and has failed to prioritize and allocate budgetary or other resources to the EBP process.[21]

In Magnet organizations, nurse engagement with EBP is highly valued, with structures and processes to support nurses to become competent with EBP; thus, Magnet organizations offer significant collaboration opportunities where librarians can play a crucial role. The evidence-based competencies for nurses set forth by Melnyk and colleagues provide a clear set of skills that nurses must have to be effective in EBP. These twenty-four competencies are set forth with thirteen core competencies for all registered nurses and include eleven more advanced competencies intended for advanced practice nurses.[22] These competencies provide librarians with a clear outline of the skills nurses need and provide librarians with the ability to identify where they can be involved to help grow the number of nurses within the organization who are competent in EBP.

VCU Health is like many other Magnet organizations in that questioning practice and finding solutions is central to nursing practice. In this environment, there are approximately one hundred evidence-based and performance-improvement projects being carried out by nurses at any one time. These projects originate from three main sources: bedside nurses initiated through a clinical ladder or unit-based initiatives, such as the Interns and Scholars or Quality Academy programs, and the Nurse Residency Program for new graduate nurses. First, there are projects initiated by experienced nurses as part of a unit-based issue or concern. Second, projects originate from the Interns and Scholars Program (ISP), which is a two-year program for experienced nurses. The program aims to improve patient care by giving practicing nurses dedicated time and resources to identify and implement an evidence-based project. Nurses may apply to the program to conduct an EBP project from question development to implementation while receiving education and support throughout the research process. Each year five to ten nurses participate in the program. The organization's third source of EBP projects is the nurse residency program (NRP), a yearlong new nurse transition to practice program with four cohorts per year. Each cohort contains approximately one hundred new graduate nurses from every hospital unit and provides the most significant number of evidence-based projects. In the program, nurse residents work individually or in a group to identify a clinical question and review the evidence for an EBP project. There are many opportunities for librarians to be involved, as the work addressing EBP aligns directly with the Magnet NK Standards. These opportunities are often done as part of the education provided across the organization, making partnering with nurse educators a natural collaboration.

The major areas where librarians can play a role are identifying practice issues through reviewing the literature, identifying practice issues, creating a clinical question, uncovering internal and external evidence, and critically appraising the evidence. Creating a clear clinical question is a multi-step process where librarians can play a key role by helping nurses think through their ideas and determine which practice issues may be ripe for practice change. This process of clarifying the question may lead to the librarian linking the nurse with organizational and subject matter experts beyond the library and helping them identify both internal and external evidence to ensure that the practice in question has the potential to be addressed. The librarian will also ensure that the clinical question is formulated clearly as part of this process. Librarians are well positioned to be an asset in this aspect of the EBP process due to librarianship training and education on information literacy, including information organization and search building. Part of that set of skills when it comes to being information literate is asking a clear question that can be used to search for information. This search for information or evidence is also where tools like the PICO format will come into play. This format allows one to break a clinical question into its key concepts, which can be used to create an effective search strategy. The structure breaks down a clinical question into its key components and makes database searching more efficient. The PICO components are P (Patient, Population, or Problem), I (Intervention), C (Comparison), and O (Outcome). With the question formulated and broken into the essential components, the search for evidence truly falls within the skill set of librarians. Librarians can help nurses identify the best databases and other resources to find evidence addressing the well-formulated clinical question. As part of this task, librarians also help with how to best search databases and utilize the limits to uncover the best-quality evidence. In the EBP process, librarians can also play a role in the critical appraisal of evidence, which may be a new skill for nurses who have not had formal training in research or EBP. Due to the amount of literature and evidence available, the ability to critically appraise findings or provide training on critical appraisal is a value-add that librarians provide to the EBP process.

The last place librarians can provide further support for the NK standards is in disseminating successful EBP initiatives. Librarians are well positioned to help nurses understand the process of writing abstracts for conferences and manuscripts. While doing this, librarians can discuss and consult or teach about the different issues that concern publishing, like copyright, choosing an appropriate journal, open-access issues, and authorship principles. While supporting dissemination, the library can also be a home for institutional repositories where posters, papers, and presentations that the nurses have authored in the organization can be housed, shared, and discovered by others interested in nursing practice topics. Additionally, not every EBP initiative will make it to publication. Still, librarians are well positioned to create internal dissemination platforms to communicate successful EBP initiatives, such as the institutional repository where these items can be discovered by others outside of the institution and help improve patient care. For example, at VCU Health, the medical librarian, with the support of VCU Libraries, set up a special collection for nurses to submit their scholarly products, and it has become increasingly popular. Repository metrics have enabled nurse authors to see that others are interested in their work. It has also allowed some to connect with nurses at other institutions and find ways to improve patient care.

An example of how the librarian could assist VCU Health during its third Magnet redesignation in 2015 included a specific EBP initiative in collaboration with nurse educators and clinicians involved in the process. As part of the collaboration around educating nurses about EBP at VCU Health, the medical librarian and collaborators noticed several areas of improvement identified. Those issues were:

- Confusion in the difference between EBP, performance improvement, and research;

- Misuse of the term "EBP project" when referring to projects using evidence, like performance improvement projects;
- Identifying topics or sources of EBP projects;
- Formulating a searchable clinical question; and
- Finding and evaluating evidence.

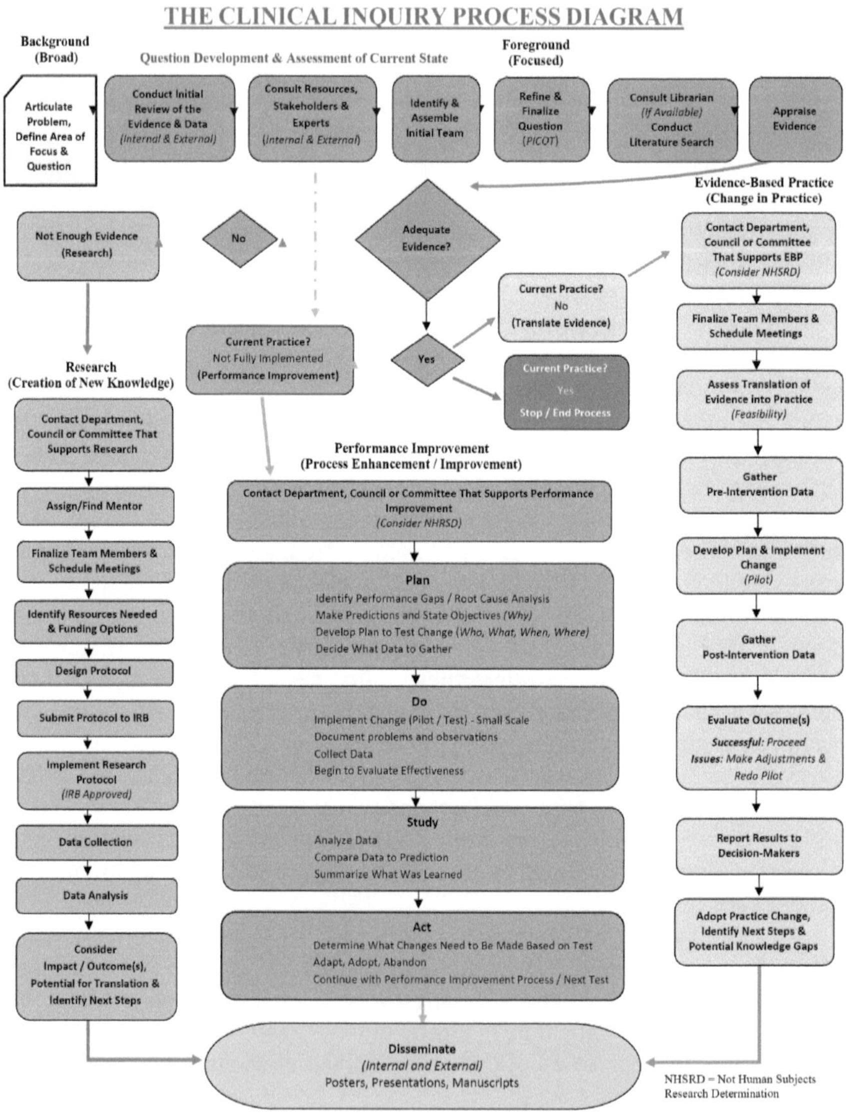

Figure 5.2. Ongoing Accreditation Efforts: Magnet Recognition and the Role of the Librarian

SOURCE: ROY BROWN

In 2009, VCU Health nurses adopted the Johns Hopkins EBP model to provide a framework for conducting all EBP initiatives. To supplement this model, the librarian, in consultation with nurses, created the Clinical Inquiry Process Diagram (see figure 5.2).[23]

This diagram provides an algorithm-like representation of the clinical inquiry process. As part of this diagram, the differences between research, EBP, and performance/quality improvement were delineated. This diagram was then used to create the Evidence-Based Practice Portfolio (EBPP) Tool, which provided just-in-time instruction for those involved in EBP initiatives. By getting nurses to use the tool and diagram, the librarian was able to help provide a consistent structure to EBP instruction. This effort resulted in nurses showing improvement in their self-reported attitudes, knowledge, and use of EBP.[24] The nurses of VCU Health adopted the diagram as part of their professional practice in 2017 around the NK standards. It provided a foundational framework for the Nursing Shared Governance Council on Clinical Inquiry and Innovations. It has been used to help standardize education, identify where resources are needed, and reshape how clinical inquiry activities are carried out.

Aside from directly assisting with EBP initiatives within the organization, librarians can also play other roles in supporting healthcare organizations pursuing Magnet Recognition. This support can occur by serving as a connecting agent between people, resources, and organization experts. Librarians base much of their work on relationships and collaborations with nurses and other organization members. Based on their work, librarians are often aware of the resources available throughout the organization. The librarian may also be aware of people or groups in the organizations who may be knowledgeable about a particular topic or engaged in research on a topic. These individuals or groups could serve as a resource to help others. Unfortunately, in many healthcare organizations, groups may work in silos and are not always aware of what others are doing (see figure 5.3).

Part of this ability to connect with others is identifying influential members within the organization, like the chief nursing officer and other leaders such as nursing directors or administrators. These individuals can help librarians serve on various committees and councils where the librarian can understand what challenges nurses are facing and where potential opportunities might be to become involved. In attending these meetings, librarians need to not only be present but also show initiative. It may not always be evident to nursing leadership what role librarians can play. Therefore, the librarian should be proactive and find ways to identify places where their value can be demonstrated. These value-added activities could be as simple as taking the initiative to provide information on a particular practice or topic before being asked. It could also involve setting up search alerts on these topics of interest and keeping nursing administrators

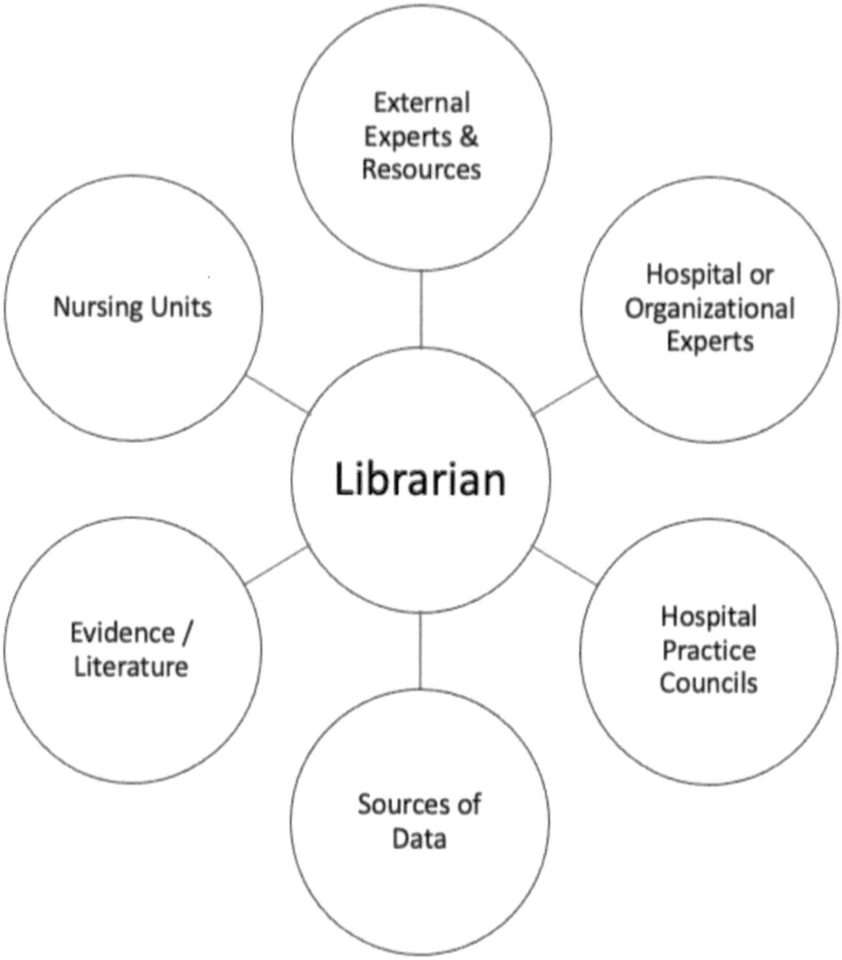

Figure 5.3. Librarian as Connecting Agent
SOURCE: ROY BROWN

aware of other activities related to using evidence to inform practice. The more value a librarian can demonstrate, the more allies a librarian can gain in an organization to do more.

CONCLUSION

The Magnet Recognition provides many opportunities for libraries and librarians to become involved and to make a meaningful contribution to healthcare research and nursing practice. This is especially true in reference to the NK Standards where EBP, research, and performance improvement initiatives are a major focus. Within this Magnet standard, librarians have specialized skills to help nurses shape their clinical questions, find appropriate evidence, appraise the evidence found, and help with the dissemination of successful EBP initiatives. In the course of this work, librarians can also support the effort by serving on committees and councils where collaborations with various individuals in nursing leadership may lead to more opportunities to contribute and get involved. In those instances where the medical librarian is a part of an academic institution, the librarian may also serve as a bridge between the academic and health system partnership. Often, the librarian who serves the nurses in the hospital may also serve the school of nursing or know the medical librarian who does. Through the support of EBP, there may also be opportunities to partner with the school of nursing faculty on EBP instruction for both the health system and the school of nursing.

Supporting these initiatives around the NK standards is also a way for the library and librarians to demonstrate value. By utilizing descriptive statistics, a librarian may show an increase in consultation or search requests for EBP projects. In addition, through their support of EBP, librarians show a return on investment if their work can be tied to improving the quality and safety outcomes like decreasing length of stay, thirty-day readmission rates, and other quality indicators.

To effectively support Magnet Recognition, librarians must actively seek opportunities to learn more about the process and what their organizations need when it comes to library services and resources. Library administration must also be willing to invest to ensure that librarians can participate in workshops and other educational opportunities to better understand the various aspects of the clinical inquiry process, whether that be in reference to evidence-based practice, research, or quality improvement. These topics are not adequately addressed in university library programs, so many librarians are ill equipped to participate fully in supporting the needs of nurses in a Magnet organization without additional professional development. In addition, evidence-based initiatives in the clinical setting have legal and human implications, underscoring the need for adequate training. Finally, libraries must invest in training for librarians to support healthcare-driven efforts that could provide long-term benefits for patients and communities.

At VCU Health, the medical librarian involved with nurses has participated fully in two Magnet redesignation cycles in both practice and acknowledgment in SOE, has participated in the Magnet site visit, and has been acknowledged as a key resource within the NK domain. The librarian's involvement has increased the utilization of the library by nurses over time and led to the health system increasing library funding based on that involvement. It has also resulted in the librarian collaborating on projects to improve evidence utilization in the hospital. Those collaborations have enabled the medical librarian to attend the ANCC National Magnet Conference and other conferences, webinars, and dissemination venues. A critical factor in this success was the support and resources utilized to build the medical librarian's skill and understanding of EBP. This minimal investment resulted in high organizational impact. It should be considered across organizations to increase visibility and recognition through specialty designations, improve healthcare teams' work environment, and promote positive outcomes for patients and communities.

ACKNOWLEDGMENTS

Author RB would like to thank Dr. Deb Zimmermann and Dr. Lauren Goodloe for their visionary leadership and support for the collaboration between nursing and the library. In addition, the authors would like to acknowledge the efforts of the VCU Health Nursing Shared Governance, Research, and Evidence-Based Practice, and Leadership Council members in the development of the Clinical Inquiry Model, figure 5.2; their input was invaluable. We would also like to recognize the Magnet expertise and leadership of Veronica Nolden, MS, RN, NEA-BC, VCU Health Patient Care Services, Professional Practice Manager, and Magnet Program Director.

NOTES

1. US Bureau of Labor Statistics, "Registered Nurses: Occupational Outlook Handbook," n.d., https://www.bls.gov/ooh/healthcare/registered-nurses.htm.
2. American Nurses Association, "Nurse Staffing Crisis: Practice & Advocacy," 2021, https://www.nursingworld.org/practice-policy/nurse-staffing/nurse-staffing-crisis/.
3. Vicki A. Lundmark, "Magnet Environments for Professional Nursing Practice," in *Patient Safety and Quality: An Evidence-Based Handbook for Nurses*, ed. Vicki A. Lundmark and Ronda G. Hughes (Rockville, MD: Agency for Healthcare Research and Quality, 2008), http://www.ncbi.nlm.nih.gov/pubmed/21328767.
4. Margaret L. McClure et al., *Magnet Hospitals: Attraction and Retention of Professional Nurses. American Academy of Nursing. Task Force on Nursing Practice in Hospitals*, American Nurses Association Publications, 1983, https://pubmed.ncbi.nlm.nih.gov/6551146/.
5. American Nurses Credentialing Center, "ANCC Magnet Recognition Program®," 2020, https://www.nursingworld.org/organizational-programs/magnet/.
6. American Nurses Credentialing Center, *2023 Magnet Application Manual* (American Nurses Credentialing Center, 2022).
7. American Nurses Credentialing Center, "Find a Magnet Organization," 2021, https://www.nursingworld.org/organizational-programs/magnet/find-a-magnet-organization/.
8. Zoë Slote Morris, Steven Wooding, and Jonathan Grant, "The Answer Is 17 Years, What Is the Question: Understanding Time Lags in Translational Research," *Journal of the Royal Society of Medicine* 104, no. 12 (December 2011): 510–20, https://doi.org/10.1258/jrsm.2011.110180.
9. John M. Westfall, James Mold, and Lyle Fagnan, "Practice-Based Research—'Blue Highways' on the NIH Roadmap," *JAMA* 297, no. 4 (January 2007): 403–6, https://doi.org/10.1001/jama.297.4.403.
10. Institute of Medicine, *Crossing the Quality Chasm* (Washington, DC: Institute of Medicine, 2003).

11. Institute of Medicine, *Evidence-Based Medicine and the Changing Nature of Health Care* (Washington, DC: National Academies Press, 2008).
12. Mark H. Ebell et al., "How Good Is the Evidence to Support Primary Care Practice?" *Evidence-Based Medicine* 22, no. 3 (June 2017): 88–92, https://doi.org/10.1136/ebmed-2017-110704.
13. Bernadette Mazurek Melnyk et al., "Nurses' Perceived Knowledge, Beliefs, Skills, and Needs Regarding Evidence-Based Practice: Implications for Accelerating the Paradigm Shift," *Worldviews on Evidence-Based Nursing* 1, no. 3 (2004): 185–93, https://doi.org/10.1111/j.1524-475X.2004.04024.x.
14. Diane S. Pravikoff, Annelle B. Tanner, and Susan T. Pierce, "Readiness of U.S. Nurses for Evidence-Based Practice," *American Journal of Nursing* 105, no. 9 (September 2005): 40–51; quiz 52, https://doi.org/10.1097/00000446-200509000-00025.
15. Bernice Mott et al., "Clinical Nurses' Knowledge of Evidence-Based Practice: Constructing a Framework to Evaluate a Multifaceted Intervention for Implementing EBP," *Contemporary Nurse: A Journal for the Australian Nursing Profession* 19, no. 1–2 (2005): 96–104, https://doi.org/10.5172/conu.19.1-2.96.
16. Hannele Saunders and Katri Vehvilainen-Julkunen, "The State of Readiness for Evidence-Based Practice among Nurses: An Integrative Review," *International Journal of Nursing Studies* 56 (April 2016): 128–40, https://doi.org/10.1016/j.ijnurstu.2015.10.018.
17. Bernadette Mazurek Melnyk et al., "The State of Evidence-Based Practice in US Nurses: Critical Implications for Nurse Leaders and Educators," *Journal of Nursing Administration* 42, no. 9 (September 2012): 410–17, https://doi.org/10.1097/NNA.0b013e3182664e0a.
18. Shaheen Majid et al., "Adopting Evidence-Based Practice in Clinical Decision Making: Nurses' Perceptions, Knowledge, and Barriers," *Journal of the Medical Library Association JMLA* 99, no. 3 (July 2011): 229–36, https://doi.org/10.3163/1536-5050.99.3.010.
19. Caroline E. Brown et al., "Nursing Practice, Knowledge, Attitudes and Perceived Barriers to Evidence-Based Practice at an Academic Medical Center," *Journal of Advanced Nursing* 65, no. 2 (February 2009): 371–81, https://doi.org/10.1111/j.1365-2648.2008.04878.x.
20. Bernadette Mazurek Melnyk et al., "A Study of Chief Nurse Executives Indicates Low Prioritization of Evidence-Based Practice and Shortcomings in Hospital Performance Metrics across the United States," *Worldviews on Evidence-Based Nursing* 13, no. 1 (2016): 6–14, https://doi.org/10.1111/wvn.12133.
21. Bernadette Mazurek Melnyk et al., "The Establishment of Evidence-Based Practice Competencies for Practicing Registered Nurses and Advanced Practice Nurses in Real-World Clinical Settings: Proficiencies to Improve Healthcare Quality, Reliability, Patient Outcomes, and Costs," *Worldviews on Evidence-Based Nursing* 11, no. 1 (February 2014): 5–15, https://doi.org/10.1111/wvn.12021.
22. Roy E. Brown, "The Clinical Inquiry Process Diagram," 2020, https://scholarscompass.vcu.edu/libraries_pubs/62/.
23. Roy E. Brown, "Empowering Nurses with an Online Roadmap for Evidence-Based Practice," *Journal of Hospital Librarianship* 20, no. 4 (October 2020): 309–22, https://doi.org/10.1080/15323269.2020.1819748.
24. Brown, "Empowering Nurses," 309–22.

BIBLIOGRAPHY

American Nurses Association. "Nurse Staffing Crisis: Practice & Advocacy," 2021. https://www.nursingworld.org/practice-policy/nurse-staffing/nurse-staffing-crisis/.

American Nurses Credentialing Center. "ANCC Magnet Recognition Program®," 2020. https://www.nursingworld.org/organizational-programs/magnet/.

———. *2023 Magnet Application Manual*. American Nurses Credentialing Center, 2022.

———. "Find a Magnet Organization," 2021. https://www.nursingworld.org/organizational-programs/magnet/find-a-magnet-organization/.

Brown, Caroline E., Mary A. Wickline, Laurie Ecoff, and Dale Glaser. "Nursing Practice, Knowledge, Attitudes and Perceived Barriers to Evidence-Based Practice at an Academic Medical Center." *Journal of Advanced Nursing* 65, no. 2 (February 2009): 371–81. https://doi.org/10.1111/j.1365-2648.2008.04878.x.

Brown, Roy E. "The Clinical Inquiry Process Diagram," 2020. https://scholarscompass.vcu.edu/libraries_pubs/62/.

Brown, Roy E. "Empowering Nurses with an Online Roadmap for Evidence-Based Practice." *Journal of Hospital Librarianship* 20, no. 4 (October 2020): 309–22. https://doi.org/10.1080/15323269.2020.1819748.

Ebell, Mark H., Randi Sokol, Aaron Lee, Christopher Simons, and Jessica Early. "How Good Is the Evidence to Support Primary Care Practice?" *Evidence-Based Medicine* 22, no. 3 (June 2017): 88–92. https://doi.org/10.1136/ebmed-2017-110704.

Institute of Medicine. *Crossing the Quality Chasm*. Washington, DC: Institute of Medicine, 2003.

———. *Evidence-Based Medicine and the Changing Nature of Health Care*. Washington, DC: National Academies Press, 2008.

———. "Keeping Patients Safe: Transforming the Work Environment of Nurses." Washington, DC: National Academies Press, 2005. http://www.nap.edu/catalog.php?record_id=11151.

Lundmark, Vicki A. "Magnet Environments for Professional Nursing Practice." In *Patient Safety and Quality: An Evidence-Based Handbook for Nurses*, edited by Vicki A. Lundmark and Ronda G. Hughes. Rockville, MD: Agency for Healthcare Research and Quality, 2008. http://www.ncbi.nlm.nih.gov/pubmed/21328767.

Majid, Shaheen, Schubert Foo, Brendan Luyt, Xue Zhang, Yin-Leng Theng, Yun-Ke Chang, and Intan A Mokhtar. "Adopting Evidence-Based Practice in Clinical Decision Making: Nurses' Perceptions, Knowledge, and Barriers." *Journal of the Medical Library Association: JMLA* 99, no. 3 (July 2011): 229–36. https://doi.org/10.3163/1536-5050.99.3.010.

McClure, Margaret L., M. Poulin, Margaret Sovie, M. Wandelt, et al. *Magnet Hospitals: Attraction and Retention of Professional Nurses. American Academy of Nursing. Task Force on Nursing Practice in Hospitals.* American Nurses Association Publications, 1983. https://pubmed.ncbi.nlm.nih.gov/6551146/.

Melnyk, Bernadette Mazurek, Ellen Fineout-Overholt, Nancy Fischbeck Feinstein, Hong Li, Leigh Small, Larry Wilcox, and Rachel Kraus. "Nurses' Perceived Knowledge, Beliefs, Skills, and Needs Regarding Evidence-Based Practice: Implications for Accelerating the Paradigm Shift." *Worldviews on Evidence-Based Nursing* 1, no. 3 (2004): 185–93. https://doi.org/10.1111/j.1524-475X.2004.04024.x.

Melnyk, Bernadette Mazurek, Ellen Fineout-Overholt, Lynn Gallagher-Ford, and Louise Kaplan. "The State of Evidence-Based Practice in US Nurses: Critical Implications for Nurse Leaders and Educators." *Journal of Nursing Administration* 42, no. 9 (September 2012): 410–17. https://doi.org/10.1097/NNA.0b013e3182664e0a.

Melnyk, Bernadette Mazurek, Lynn Gallagher-Ford, Lisa English Long, and Ellen Fineout-Overholt. "The Establishment of Evidence-Based Practice Competencies for Practicing Registered Nurses and Advanced Practice Nurses in Real-World Clinical Settings: Proficiencies to Improve Healthcare Quality, Reliability, Patient Outcomes, and Costs." *Worldviews on Evidence-Based Nursing* 11, no. 1 (February 2014): 5–15. https://doi.org/10.1111/wvn.12021.

Melnyk, Bernadette Mazurek, Lynn Gallagher-Ford, Bindu Koshy Thomas, Michelle Troseth, Kathy Wyngarden, and Laura Szalacha. "A Study of Chief Nurse Executives Indicates Low Prioritization of Evidence-Based Practice and Shortcomings in Hospital Performance Metrics across the United States." *Worldviews on Evidence-Based Nursing* 13, no. 1 (2016): 6–14. https://doi.org/10.1111/wvn.12133.

Morris, Zoë Slote, Steven Wooding, and Jonathan Grant. "The Answer Is 17 Years, What Is the Question: Understanding Time Lags in Translational Research." *Journal of the Royal Society of Medicine* 104, no. 12 (December 2011): 510–20. https://doi.org/10.1258/jrsm.2011.110180.

Mott, Bernice, Joanne Nolan, Nadia Zarb, Vanessa Arnison, Roxan Chan, Tracey Codner, Therese Casey, et al. "Clinical Nurses' Knowledge of Evidence-Based Practice: Constructing a Framework to Evaluate a Multifaceted Intervention for Implementing EBP." *Contemporary Nurse: A Journal for the Australian Nursing Profession* 19, no. 1-2 (2005): 96-104. https://doi.org/10.5172/conu.19.1-2.96.

Pravikoff, Diane S., Annelle B. Tanner, and Susan T. Pierce. "Readiness of U.S. Nurses for Evidence-Based Practice." *American Journal of Nursing* 105, no. 9 (September 2005): 40–51; quiz 52. https://doi.org/10.1097/00000446-200509000-00025.

Saunders, Hannele, and Katri Vehvilainen-Julkunen. "The State of Readiness for Evidence-Based Practice among Nurses: An Integrative Review." *International Journal of Nursing Studies* 56 (April 2016): 128–40. https://doi.org/10.1016/j.ijnurstu.2015.10.018.

US Bureau of Labor Statistics. "Registered Nurses: Occupational Outlook Handbook," n.d. https://www.bls.gov/ooh/healthcare/registered-nurses.htm.

Westfall, John M., James Mold, and Lyle Fagnan. "Practice-Based Research—'Blue Highways' on the NIH Roadmap." *JAMA* 297, no. 4 (January 2007): 403–6. https://doi.org/10.1001/jama.297.4.403.

6

Making a Continuous Impact

LIBRARY PARTICIPATION IN THE CONTINUOUS QUALITY IMPROVEMENT PROCESS

Charlotte M. Beyer, Rosalind Franklin University

WHY IS ACCREDITATION IMPORTANT IN HEALTH SCIENCES EDUCATION?

Accreditation is defined as a formal evaluation by a third party to determine if an organization has met a certain standard of excellence and quality and is therefore qualified to carry out certain tasks.[1] Accreditation occurs across a variety of disciplines and organizations, from hospitals to zoos to manufacturing. Accreditation assures people outside the organizations that the organization in question meets at least certain minimum standards in terms of quality assurance. Two industries where confirmation of quality assurance is critical are healthcare organizations and higher education institutions. Combining elements of these two industries are healthcare training programs. Accreditation in health professions education is critical; on top of ensuring a quality educational experience, a health professions education and training program needs to constantly improve due to the changing needs of the healthcare workforce.[2] Improving the educational experience in terms of didactic and experiential learning not only has the potential to improve the experience for the student but also has the potential to move the industry of healthcare forward and improve the health of future patients with new discoveries and innovations.[3]

Accreditation pushes health professions training to constantly improve and self-reflect on educational and training practices, ensuring the graduates have the tools to not only function in healthcare environments like hospitals and clinics but provide the best possible care and innovate as things change. One example is the innovations that are needed in global health crises such as the COVID-19 pandemic. Health sciences education is the base or foundation for clinical practice, which is always changing and stressed. Healthcare is also a team-based activity; everyone has a role in the success of a team. In higher education, there is no place that is better seen as the accreditation process. It can be said that accreditation is one of the most important forms of teamwork higher education institutions complete. Everyone has a role to play in the success of the team across the university, which is why the library is a critical component in any accreditation process: we are experts in providing access and education around information, which is the foundation of the educational experience.

WHAT IS CONTINUOUS QUALITY IMPROVEMENT?

Continuous Quality Improvement (CQI) is defined as a structured process for constantly assessing internal processes while implementing improvements with the goal of providing high-quality outcomes. It is important to note that this process is proactive rather than reactive and that in healthcare the improvements are made with the goal of improving the outcomes for patients, from improving overall care to reducing costs by maximizing efficiency.[4] CQI is considered a best practice in many different disciplines in healthcare due to the changing nature of healthcare as an industry.[5] In terms of healthcare training and educational programs, over the past few years, CQI has come to the

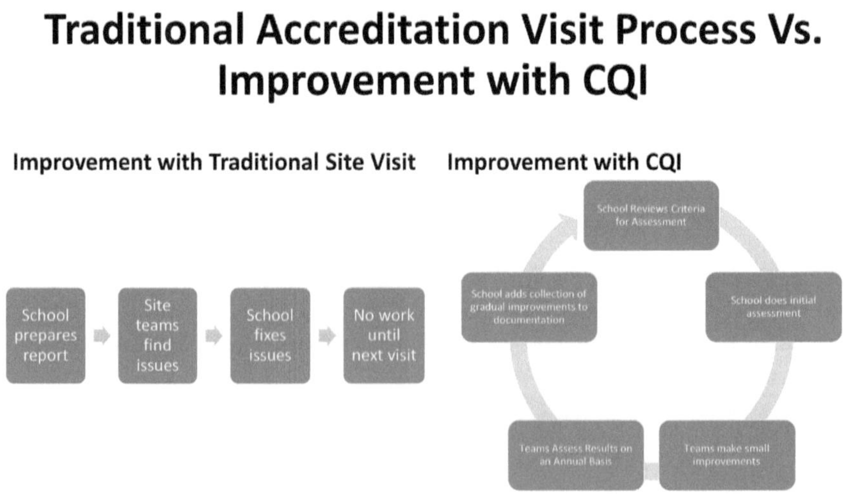

Figure 6.1. Traditional Accreditation Visit Process Vs. Improvement with CQI
SOURCE: CHARLOTTE M. BEYER

forefront of importance; many have recognized the importance of always evaluating and improving in order to cultivate a healthcare workforce that meets not only current needs but future ones as well.[6,7] Many different accrediting bodies have adopted CQI, but the one that will be highlighted in this chapter in particular is the LCME, which accredits institutions for medical education. Figure 6.1 shows the difference between Traditional Accreditation Visit and CQI in Accreditation.

LCME stands for the Liaison Committee on Medical Education, which is cosponsored by the Association of American Medical Colleges (AAMC) and the American Medical Association (AMA). This is the accrediting body for all allopathic-medicine medical schools in the United States and Canada. Like many other accrediting bodies, LCME has a structured multi-stage process for awarding accreditation to prospective institutions. These institutions must demonstrate to LCME that their program meets a set of educational and program-related standards set by LCME.[8] The standards and their sub-elements cover everything from didactic education, clinical rotation placements, student life and extracurriculars, faculty development, and more.[9] There are three main stages of the accreditation: preliminary, provisional, and full status. Institutions must provide documentation of how the individual institutions translated/plan to translate the LCME standards and elements into practice. This documentation comes in the form of written documentation as well as in live interviews with key stakeholders during site visits. Since the library is a key partner in supporting curriculum development, the library team is involved at every stage of the accreditation process. Contributions from members of the library team include shaping the documentation sent to LCME and participating in the interviews during the in-person site visits.[10] Once a medical school is awarded full accreditation, LCME will provide a time frame for another site visit to occur, to assess continued adherence to the LCME standards. The amount of time between visits is dependent on how the school performed at the previous site visit, with typically a maximum of eight years between visits. Once a school moves into a regular cycle of site visits after being awarded full status, there are two critical documents that must be updated before the next visit. These two documents are the self-study and the DCI, or Data Collection Instrument, which utilize the twelve LCME standards. Since the library provides resources and services that impact a variety of areas, members of the library team contribute to multiple standards documented in the DCI and the self-study.

The LCME adjusted the standards around 2015 to include a CQI element in the first standard that is focused on mission, planning, organization, and integrity.[11] Specifically, it required that programs describe the CQI processes that their institution uses to establish both the short- and long-term programmatic goals. To emphasize the importance of CQI within medical education, LCME made it the first element of the first standard.[12] A primary reason for adjusting the standards was to take a more proactive approach to identifying and improving issues prior to the survey visit. Prior to 2015, medical schools would typically get a report of the areas of noncompliance, there would be a follow-up visit, and LCME would review concerns to determine whether they were resolved. If LCME assessed that their concerns were addressed, the school would not have to take further action until the next review.[13] The goal of embedding CQI in the site visit process was to encourage schools to develop a culture of self-reflection and to continually identify areas of standard compliance as well as areas of improvement.[14] With the traditional model, which was reactive, there is only so much time to change and improve things before the visit. With CQI, self-reflection and assessment are built into the process for a more structured and deeper level of improvement.[15] One of the hallmarks for an effective QI process to be successful is the work of a team with a variety of voices and perspectives.[16] This means not only medical school faculty but also student perspectives and units like the library that support the medical school. It is important to note that since it is a process that needs to be tailored to the institution to meet its unique needs, LCME did not dictate exactly how CQI should be implemented at each individual school; it was up to the institutions themselves to determine how it should be done and to report on it in the DCI. Due to its inclusion as an official element, many medical schools began implementing CQI at their institutions in a variety of ways.[17]

CQI AT CHICAGO MEDICAL SCHOOL AND THE LIBRARY'S ROLE

CHICAGO MEDICAL SCHOOL (CMS) AT ROSALIND FRANKLIN UNIVERSITY OF MEDICINE AND SCIENCE (RFUMS)

The next part of this chapter describes the library's involvement in the CQI process established in the Chicago Medical School (CMS) for the Allopathic Medicine program at Rosalind Franklin University of Medicine and Science (RFUMS). RFUMS is a private, graduate interprofessional health sciences university located in North Chicago, Illinois, which is halfway between Milwaukee and Chicago. RFUMS currently has six colleges: the Chicago Medical School, College of Health Professions, College of Nursing, College of Pharmacy, School of Graduate and Postdoctoral Studies, and William M. Scholl College of Podiatric Medicine. In terms of how medical schools are categorized by the AAMC, CMS is considered a community-based school, which means there is not an integrated teaching hospital associated with the medical school. Often with these types of schools, clinical education is done in collaboration with community hospitals as clinical partners rather than academic medical centers where the hospital and medical school are under the same institution.[18] Being community based has a few unique challenges; student experiences can vary at the clinical sites because they are not all under one umbrella like an academic medical center. This is also seen in the CQI process, because change happens at different rates at these institutions. Enrollment in the four-year allopathic program is about 800 FTE. Specifically, this section is a case study on how members of the library team are involved in accreditation activities in CMS and how being involved in these activities has shaped the library's work of supporting the curriculum and supporting the university's mission.

STANDARDS-BASED CONTINUOUS QUALITY LEADERSHIP PROJECT

In 2015, CMS started to pilot a Standards-Based Continuous Quality Leadership (SBCQL) project that would begin to develop a CQI process at CMS. The SBCQL project was constructed so that each standard would have a lead who would organize the work for their team and identify key partners who would be invited to their teams. As noted, the goal of CQI is team based and requires expertise from many different stakeholders from not only CMS but the university at large. The leads would gather once a month and present on their standard. Since there were twelve standards and twelve months in the year, standard 1 would present in January with standard 12 presenting in December and each standard giving an annual report in their month. The focus when the project started was establishing what was considered in compliance and what would be examples of excellence for each element in the LCME standards. To start to gather this data, the standard leads' first project was to fill out a dashboard in an Excel format that listed each standard and each element within that standard. Each standard team directed their standard leads to complete what a standard of compliance and a standard of excellence would look like. Types of benchmarking data would be identified to be used as evidence if an element met compliance and excellence. This benchmarking data would also be used to determine an overall rating for the element by color, with blue being excellent, green being something that needed to be improved, and yellow being deficient. In addition to benchmarking data, the element leads would also include narratives. If something was below a blue, a narrative for moving the element to the next level was suggested. Individual standard teams would meet and then discuss narratives in the dashboard with the ratings applied to those elements. Element leads would receive feedback on their work with not only ways to improve the narrative but ideas for moving elements up in the rating system, with the goal of moving as many elements to blue status as possible. The rating and suggestions would then be presented in the yearly presentation for discussion by the element leads. In 2015–2018 the focus was on the dashboard and getting that in order; that information was used to prepare for the DCI as the site visit preparation time approached.

BOXER LIBRARY TEAM AND ROLE IN THE SBCQL PROJECT

The Boxer Library is the sole library that serves and supports all academic programs within the six colleges at RFUMS. The library team consists of eight team members and includes four librarians and four professional staff. Each person has an area of expertise from instruction to electronic resources to access and technical services. Multiple members of the team are called upon in the accreditation process in relation to their areas of expertise. For example, the electronic resources librarian might advise on the number of electronic serials in the collection, while the instruction and reference librarian may contribute instruction numbers. Coordination of who contributes what to the different accreditation activities is the responsibility of the library director, who is the primary point of contact for academic programs and the library. The library director then assigns staff with appropriate levels of expertise to accreditation tasks as they become available, taking into consideration not only the expertise but the workload of the employee.

In 2015, the library was invited to participate in the pilot of the SBCQL project; the three positions that were directly involved in the SBCQL teams were the library director, instruction and reference librarian, and electronic resources librarian. Within the twelve accreditation standards identified by LCME that would be in the dashboard and later DCI, the library was involved in two different standards. These standards are Standard 5: Educational Resources and Infrastructure and Standard 6: Competencies, Curricular Objectives, and Curricular Design. In each of these standards, a library team member served as element lead for a portion of the standard. These were Element 5.8: Library Resources and Staff and Element 6.3: Self-Directed and Life-Long Learning. The library team had a few roles in the beginning of the project. Toward the beginning of the project, the library director was asked to be the lead not only for Element 5.8: Library Resources and Staff but for Standard 5: Educational Resources and Infrastructure as well. The library director fulfilled that role from 2015 to 2020, before stepping down to allow a faculty member from the medical school to take on that role. At the point the library director retained the prior to the SBCQL project, the library director was appointed an adviser to the CMS curriculum committee and therefore had an established presence for advising on the use of educational resources in the curriculum. In addition to serving as an expert in the acquisition of resources, the library director also served as an advocate for library involvement in embedding evidence-based medicine (EBM) within the curriculum. EBM is a decision-making process that integrates knowledge gained through clinical experience, patient values, and best available evidence in literature.[19] In addition to providing expertise in information retrieval to support EBM, many librarians are now providing additional expertise in the critical appraisal practices needed to assess the quality of that literature. Librarians defining best practices for critical appraisal has been tied to lifelong and self-directed learning. Within the LCME standards, Standard 6.3: Self-Directed and Life-Long Learning focuses on these concepts within the larger element 6: Competencies, Curricular Objectives, and Curricular Design. Since LCME introduced this sub-element as a key part of the standards, medical schools started to look for ways to ensure students met these competencies. Since librarians are key experts in the process of teaching how to find and appraise information, it resulted in librarians being involved in designing self-directed learning activities to meet this standard.[20] Initially, the library director was asked to participate as the Standard 6.3: Self-Directed and Life-Long Learning lead. In 2017, the element lead role was transferred to the instruction and reference librarian, who was leading the instructional activities of the library. Having the library in multiple elements was a big benefit, as the library was able to have multiple voices in relation to library impact in the CMS curriculum, which led to a better understanding of the role of the library in the educational experience of the students in the medical school. Significant benefits to participating in this process will be discussed in the next section of the chapter.

LIBRARY INVOLVEMENT IN CQI RELATED TO ACCREDITATION: A ROADMAP

The next part of the chapter will outline a roadmap for libraries participating in a CQI process related to accreditation. This roadmap will provide examples from the experience of the Boxer Library team in the CMS SBCQL project and the maps in a cycle; it is a continuous process. There are four main parts of this roadmap: identifying benchmarks, using benchmark data to tell a story, assessing benchmarking data, and using benchmark data for assessment and improvement. Once the roadmap has been started, it is a cycle; the assessment might lead to new benchmarks, which starts the cycle again. Each point on the roadmap will have

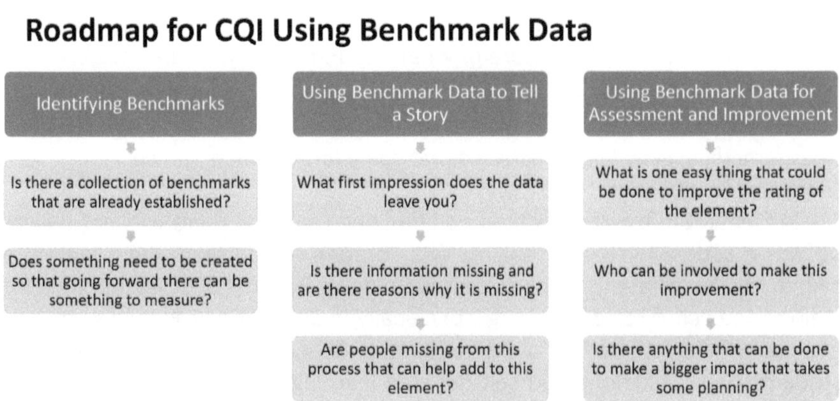

Figure 6.2. Roadmap for CQI Using Benchmark Data
SOURCE: CHARLOTTE M. BEYER

a few clarifying questions to help a library team meet that need. This roadmap can be viewed in figure 6.2.

IDENTIFYING BENCHMARKS

The first step in the roadmap is the process of identifying benchmarks that will be used in the CQI process. Think of this as the foundation that a house will be built upon. When selecting benchmarking, a few things need to be considered, which can be defined in a few questions.

IDENTIFYING BENCHMARKS QUESTIONS

- Is there a collection of already established benchmarks that are of value to the unit working in the accreditation process?
- If there is not a clear definitive source for benchmarking, does something need to be created so that going forward there can be something to measure?
- What is the value for the benchmarks in terms of compliance and excellence?

Is there an established collection of benchmarks?

In this case, is there a set of established benchmarks that are important to the medical school? In the case of CMS for Element 5.8, a few surveys were already established with information about the library that held value to not only CMS but LCME as well. These resources included the Independent Student Analysis (ISA), the AAMC medical school graduation questionnaire, and internal institutional student satisfaction surveys. A combination of these three sources provided a picture of what needed to be measured for Element 5.8: Library Resources/Staff.

Does something need to be created so that going forward there can be something to measure?

In Element 6.3: Self-Directed and Life-Long Learning, there was not a clear definitive source for benchmarking. The librarian on the team did a literature search to scan what other universities were doing in terms of protected time for lifelong and self-directed learning, specifically in defining policies. This resulted in a policy being created for protected time to define how much protected time students had for lifelong and self-directed learning projects. One benefit that came out of this project was that members of the medical school saw the expertise of the librarians outside of acquisitions, because they were able to discuss the research and apply it to the curriculum. This experience ended up leading to other literature search projects for other initiatives in the medical school, with more opportunities for medical school faculty and administration to partner with librarians with the goal of creating high-quality medical education. These partnerships may have not been formed if not for the SBCQL project.

What is the value for the benchmarks in terms of compliance and excellence?

Determining at the beginning the value for the benchmarks for compliance and excellence so there is a goal to meet and/or strive for can help to frame the narrative later. For the library this meant that the library needed to meet a student satisfaction score within 5 percent of the national average for compliance and above 5 percent of the national average for excellence for the AAMC graduation questionnaire, as an example. Establishing this early on will help assess the element that comes later in the roadmap.

USING THE BENCHMARKING DATA TO TELL A STORY

Once the benchmarking data has been identified, the next step is to gather the data and use it to tell an effective story even as the narrative is in short form, like a dashboard in an Excel spreadsheet. Data by itself does not tell a lot, but woven with the context of the experiences of the medical school curriculum, it can paint a snapshot of not only how the element is viewed at the present time but also how it can be improved for the future.

ASSESSING BENCHMARKING DATA

When assessing benchmarking data for the first time, there are three main questions you should answer to tell you where you are on the benchmarking part of the CQI roadmap.

ASSESSING BENCHMARKING DATA QUESTIONS

- What first impression does the data leave you?
- Is there information missing, and are there reasons why it is missing?
- Are people missing from this process who can help add to this element?

What first impression does the data leave you?

For example, the first year the satisfaction graduation score for the library was over 90 percent, which reiterated that the students were satisfied with the overall library services. However, the next year it was lower, which led to a discussion and narrative as to why the data changed.

Is there information missing, and are there reasons why it is missing?

This process can be one that is a type of record keeping for the progression of the curriculum. For example, during the COVID-19 pandemic, scores for access to materials may be lower, and by association the scores may be lower because students are not able to access the materials. This type of information is important for the assessment. Since CQI is done annually, changes that occur one year may be different in the future. The main part of this section of the roadmap is the interpretation of the data at that time.

Are people missing from this process who can help add to this element?

In Element 6.3: Self-Directed and Life-Long Learning, the instructors for case-based learning had to be consulted to see how they incorporated case-based learning and how self-directed learning intersects with those cases. That discussion led to other discussions about what self-directed learning is, and how evidence-based medicine could be incorporated into it. This also led to discussions about librarian expertise to possibly support self-directed learning as well. This further helped to develop the parameters for the protected time policy and the importance of self-directed learning.

USING THE BENCHMARKING DATA FOR ASSESSMENT AND IMPROVEMENT

Once the data's story has been told, the final step is to assess what was found and how the data could be used to improve for the future. The point of using the benchmarking data is to not only assess what currently exists but to identify improvements for the future to ensure a high-quality educational experience.

Assessing Benchmarking Data Questions

- What is one easy thing that could be done to improve the rating of the element?
- Who can be involved to make this improvement?
- What can be done to make a bigger impact that takes some planning?

What is one easy thing that could be done to improve the rating of the element?

For example, in Element 5.8, the student satisfaction score indicated that students were most unhappy with the journal coverage, so the library did some research about accessing journal articles in a few courses; the scores improved the next year. During the COVID-19 pandemic there were comments about access to materials; education about Interlibrary Loan was also included.

Who can be involved to make this improvement?

Who is involved in the improvement process is important because effective partnerships are vital to making things work. One tool that some medical schools use to track improvements in areas first identified by students is a "You Said, We Did" document. This document will list in the form of a website or handout areas of concern or suggestions raised by the students and then a bullet point with the action the college took to address that concern or suggestion. This is a wonderful tool to use, especially when an area of concern can be improved through education to directly connect with the students. Figure 6.3 provides an example of what a "You Said, We Did" document could look like.

What can be done to make a bigger impact that takes some planning?

In Element 5.8, one place for improvement was the types of study spaces available to the students. The library took that information and created new

You Said	We Did
It would be helpful to have an online chat service to answer library questions.	The library team launched an online chat service staffed by librarians 9:00am - 4:00pm, Monday-Friday.
There are not enough electrical outlets for student devices in the quiet area of the library.	The library team worked with facilities to install more electrical outlets in the quiet area as well as investing in more surge protectors.
Students need to charge their devices before tests, and often forget their chargers.	The library team purchased phone and laptop chargers for checkout at the Circulation Desk.
Students are overwhelmed by email with all the announcements on campus.	The library team launched a quarterly newsletter to coordinate announcing in one email instead of sending out multiple email each quarter.
Students want more standup desks to study on in the library.	The library team partnered with the Department of Student Wellness to purchase 5 new standing desks for the library spaces.

Figure 6.3. Example of You Said, We Did
SOURCE: CHARLOTTE M. BEYER

modern study spaces for the students to use. Using information from the CQI projects helped prioritize projects within the university. These improvements could then be tracked in the following year's entry into the dashboard. This would then turn into a narrative for the DCI that would be one of the building blocks for the accreditation site visit.

USING THE INFORMATION FROM CQI PROJECTS TO GUIDE LIBRARY POLICIES AND PROCEDURES

One way that CQI can be used in library operations is the creation and maintenance of annual reports and documentation. Like CQI projects, annual reports can create a snapshot of how the library is performing and where it is going in the future. One of the main assessment questions in libraries is how to start and what to assess. The benchmarking data can provide answers to those questions by providing starting points for conversations as well as topics to revisit year after year. For example, some of the data found in the SBCQL projects helped to inform the types of information that the library needed to track for its own internal assessment. The library currently has its own dashboard with data that is updated annually. This dashboard is the basis of the library director's annual presentation on how the library has been doing and where it is going. When creating an annual report, questions that the library team asks are: what were the top takeaways from the SBCQL project and how can we translate it to our dashboard statistics and then use it to help benchmarking in the future? The ISA, Graduation Questionnaire, and internal student satisfaction surveys all have questions related to library spaces, resources, and services in some ways. Some of the questions include:

Please rate your experience related to the library on campus.

- Library hours are adequate for my study needs.
- Library staff are helpful, responsive, and approachable.

- I have adequate access to databases and collections in the library.

The library looked at the data from the survey and then brainstormed how to improve for the future. This was a combination of both education on the library's part and brainstorming services for the future. In terms of the annual report, the library answered the question of access to resources by showing the number of hits to library resources and the use of interlibrary loan in a year. One other improvement that came out of the CQI process and maintenance of the dashboard was the release of an online chat service in March 2020. That service came to be when the library staff looked at the scores from the satisfaction questionnaires and tried to think of ways to meet students where they are located. One suggestion that came from the student library advisory committee was for an online chat service for reference questions. In March 2020, the online chat service was launched to keep in contact with students during the first stage of the coronavirus pandemic.[21] The library then used the data from the online chat service in the dashboard to communicate how the library responded to students in 2020. Figure 6.4 shows an image of one of the slides from the dashboard.

That information can be used in the dashboard as an example of measures the library took to improve services in the CQI process to support questions around staff assistance in the various surveys. By using the benchmarking data sources as a framework for assessing resources and services, the library can continually respond to student needs and improve as changes arise.

CONCLUSION

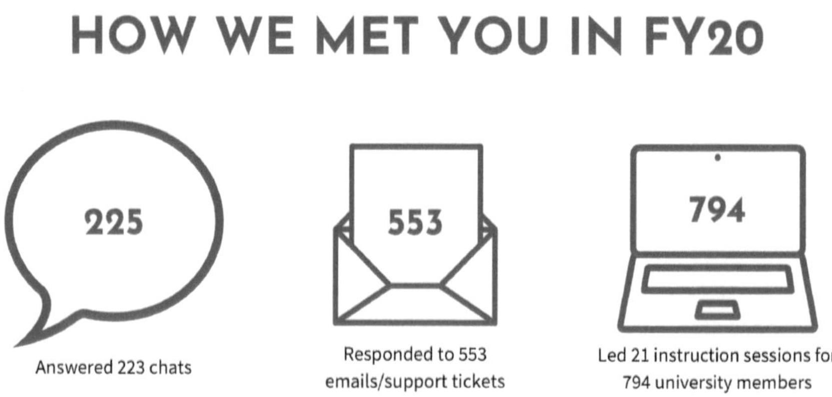
HOW WE MET YOU IN FY20
225
553
794
Answered 223 chats
Responded to 553
emails/support tickets
Led 21 instruction sessions for
794 university members

Figure 6.4. Dashboard Slide for How We Met You in 2020
SOURCE: CHARLOTTE M.BEYER

This chapter provides an overview of what continuous quality improvement is, how it intersects with accreditation, and how libraries can involve themselves in the process to improve their own processes while creating partnerships, which moves both the library and institution forward. The healthcare field is always in a state of constant change with new innovations and discoveries, which is why CQI thrives. The main goal of using CQI is to promote a growth mindset where fields can evolve to the needs of participants and stakeholders. In medical education, this results in adapting best practices and educational competencies to the current needs of future healthcare professionals. Medical best practices will continually change throughout graduates' careers, so the goal of medical education is to provide the roots or the foundation that graduates can grow from as they gain clinical expertise. One of the best ways is to have a growth mindset with CQI so faculty and staff can meet students where they are and adapt to their needs as they change. Like healthcare, librarianship is an evolving field that is constantly changing and needs to evolve as the environment changes. By answering the questions presented in the roadmap, library teams can not only add to the CQI process in accreditation but can also use some of the same questions as they assess their own services in a continuous improvement model.

ACKNOWLEDGMENTS

The Boxer Library's involvement in the SBCQL project was due to the hard work of many people at RFUMS. Specifically, the author would like to thank Scott Thomson, who was library director when the SBCQL was first implemented and advocated for library involvement while establishing some of the practices outlined in this chapter. The author would like to also thank faculty and staff in the Chicago Medical School for opening doors for the library to become involved in this process.

NOTES

1. International Accreditation Service, "What Is Accreditation?" accessed January 4, 2022, https://www.iasonline.org/about-ias/what-is-accreditation/.
2. World Health Organization, "Transforming and Scaling Up Health Professionals' Education And Training," 2013, https://www.who.int/publications/i/item/transforming-and-scaling-up-health-professionals%E2%80%99-education-and-training.
3. Jason R. Frank et al., "The Role of Accreditation in 21st Century Health Professions Education: Report of an International Consensus Group," *BMC Medical Education* 20 (2020): 1–9. https://doi.org/10.1186/s12909-020-02121-5. Society of Hospital Medicine, "Continuous Quality Improvement," *Journal of Hospital Medicine* 5, no. S2 (2010), https://doi.org/10.1002/jhm.764.
4. Janya McCalman et al., "Continuous Quality Improvement and Comprehensive Primary Health Care: A Systems Framework to Improve Service Quality and Health Outcomes," *Frontiers in Public Health* 6 (2018), https://www.frontiersin.org/article/10.3389/fpubh.2018.00076.

5. Matthew M. Anderson and Andrew N. Garman, "Preparing Future Healthcare Leaders through Graduate Education: Impact of Program Accreditation on Quality Improvement," *Journal of Allied Health* 47, no. 2 (2018): 121–25.

6. Barbara Barzansky et al.,, "Continuous Quality Improvement in an Accreditation System for Undergraduate Medical Education: Benefits and Challenges." *Medical Teacher* 37, no. 11 (2015): 1032–38. https://doi.org/10.3109/0142159X.2015.1031735.

7. Liaison Committee on Medical Education, "Scope and Purpose of Accreditation," accessed January 22, 2022, https://lcme.org/about/.

8. Liaison Committee on Medical Education, "Functions and Structure of a Medical School—(contains the LCME Standards)," accessed January 4, 2022, https://lcme.org/publications/.

9. Nadine Dexter et al., "Building New Twenty-First Century Medical School Libraries from the Ground Up: Challenges, Experiences, and Lessons Learned," *Journal of the Medical Library Association* 107, no. 1 (2019): 6–15, https://doi.org/10.5195/jmla.2019.493.

10. Ibid.

11. Liaison Committee on Medical Education, "LCME Accreditation," paper presented at the AAMC Learn Serve Lead 2016, http://lcme.org/wp-content/uploads/filebase/LCME-Accreditation-
A-Tool-for-Improvement_2016-11-12.pdf.

12. Ibid.

13. Ibid.

14. Brian M. Wong and Linda A. Headrick, "Application of Continuous Quality Improvement to Medical Education," *Medical Education* 55, no. 1 (2021): 72–81, https://doi.org/10.1111/medu.14351.

15. Terry D. Stratton, "Legitimizing Continuous Quality Improvement (CQI): Navigating Rationality in Undergraduate Medical Education," *JGIM: Journal of General Internal Medicine* 34, no. 5 (2019): 758–61, https://doi.org/10.1007/s11606-019-04875-1.

16. Jason S. Hedrick et al., "A Review of Continuous Quality Improvement Processes at Ten Medical Schools." *Medical Science Educator* 29, no. 1 (2019): 285–90.

17. Ibid.

18. AAMC, "Brief Definition of Fields," accessed January 4, 2022, https://www.aamc.org/data-reports/reporting-tools/brief-definition-fields.

19. David L. Sackett et al., "Evidence Based Medicine: What It Is and What It Isn't," *BMJ* 312 (1996): 71–72, https://doi.org/10.1136/bmj.312.7023.71.

20. Natalie Tagge and Jenny Pierce, "Librarians Flip Out: Leveraging Librarians' Skills to Teach Self-Directed Learning Competencies," poster presented at the Innovations in Medical Education conference, February 23–24, 2018, Los Angeles, CA, https://scholarshare.temple.edu/handle/20.500.12613/74.

21. Charlotte Beyer et al., "Developing and Sustaining a Virtual Reference Service with a Small Library Team," in *Virtual Services in the Health Sciences Library*, ed. Amanda Scull (Lanham, MD: Rowman & Littlefield, 2022).

BIBLIOGRAPHY

AAMC. "Brief Definition of Fields." Accessed January 4, 2022, https://www.aamc.org/data-reports/reporting-tools/brief-definition-fields.

Anderson, Matthew M., and Andrew N. Garman. "Preparing Future Healthcare Leaders through Graduate Education: Impact of Program Accreditation on Quality Improvement." *Journal of Allied Health* 47, no. 2 (2018): 121–25.

Barzansky, Barbara, Dan Hunt, Geneviève Moineau, Ducksun Ahn, Chi-Wan Lai, Holly Humphrey, and Linda Peterson. "Continuous Quality Improvement in an Accreditation System for Undergraduate Medical Education: Benefits and Challenges." *Medical Teacher* 37, no. 11 (2015): 1032–38. https://doi.org/10.3109/0142159X.2015.1031735.

Beyer, Charlotte, KatieRose McEneely, Claressa Slaughter, and Chelsea Eidbo. "Developing and Sustaining a Virtual Reference Service with a Small Library Team." In *Virtual Services in the Health Sciences Library*, edited by Amanda Scull. Lanham, MD: Rowman & Littlefield, 2022.

Dexter, Nadine, Joanne M. Muellenbach, Elizabeth R. Lorbeer, Debra Rand, Matthew E. Wilcox, and Bradley A. Long. "Building New Twenty-First Century Medical School Libraries from the Ground Up: Challenges, Experiences, and Lessons Learned." *Journal of the Medical Library Association* 107, no. 1 (2019): 6–15. https://doi.org/10.5195/jmla.2019.493.

Frank, Jason R., Sarah Taber, Marta van Zanten, Fedde Scheele, Danielle Blouin, and on behalf of the International Health Professions Accreditation, Outcomes Consortium. "The Role of Accreditation in 21st Century Health Professions Education: Report of an International Consensus Group." *BMC Medical Education* 20 (2020): 1–9. https://doi.org/10.1186/s12909-020-02121-5.

Hedrick, Jason S., Scott Cottrell, Debra Stark, Erica Brownfield, Hugh A. Stoddard, S. M. Angle, Lecretia A. Buckley, C. R. Clinch, Karin Esposito, N. K. Krane, Vicki Park, Cayla R. Teal, and Norman D. Ferrari III. "A Review of Continuous Quality Improvement Processes at Ten Medical Schools." *Medical Science Educator* 29, no. 1 (2019): 285–90.

International Accreditation Service. "What Is Accreditation?" Accessed January 4, 2022. https://www.iasonline.org/about-ias/what-is-accreditation/.

Liaison Committee on Medical Education. "Functions and Structure of a Medical School—(contains the LCME Standards)." Accessed January 4, 2022. https://lcme.org/publications/.

———, "LCME Accreditation." Paper presented at the AAMC Learn Serve Lead 2016. http://lcme.org/wp-content/uploads/filebase/LCME-Accreditation-A-Tool-for-Improvement_2016-11-12.pdf.

———. "Scope and Purpose of Accreditation." Accessed January 22, 2022. https://lcme.org/about/.

McCalman, Janya, Ross Bailie, Roxanne Bainbridge, Karen McPhail-Bell, Nikki Percival, Deborah Askew, Ruth Fagan, and Komla Tsey. "Continuous Quality Improvement and Comprehensive Primary Health Care: A Systems Framework to Improve Service Quality and Health Outcomes." *Frontiers in Public Health* 6 (2018). https://www.frontiersin.org/article/10.3389/fpubh.2018.00076.

Sackett, David. L., William M. C. Rosenberg, J. A. Muir Gray, R. Bryan Haynes, and W. Scott Richardson. "Evidence Based Medicine: What It Is and What It Isn't." *BMJ* 312 (1996): 71–72. https://doi.org/10.1136/bmj.312.7023.71.

Society of Hospital Medicine. "Continuous Quality Improvement." *Journal of Hospital Medicine* 5, no. S2 (2010). https://doi.org/10.1002/jhm.764.

Stratton, Terry D. "Legitimizing Continuous Quality Improvement (CQI): Navigating Rationality in Undergraduate Medical Education." *JGIM: Journal of General Internal Medicine* 34, no. 5 (2019): 758–61. https://doi.org/10.1007/s11606-019-04875-1.

Tagge, Natalie, and Jenny Pierce. "Librarians Flip Out: Leveraging Librarians' Skills to Teach Self-Directed Learning Competencies." Poster presented at the Innovations in Medical Education conference, February 23–24, 2018, Los Angeles, CA. https://scholarshare.temple.edu/handle/20.500.12613/74.

Wong, Brian M., and Linda A. Headrick. "Application of Continuous Quality Improvement to Medical Education." *Medical Education* 55, no. 1 (2021): 72–81. https://doi.org/10.1111/medu.14351.

World Health Organization. "Transforming and Scaling Up Health Professionals' Education and Training." 2013. https://www.who.int/publications/i/item/transforming-and-scaling-up-health-professionals%E2%80%99-education-and-training.

7

From the Source

COLLECTED INSIGHTS FROM ACCREDITING OFFICERS

Darell Schmick, John J. Dougherty, and Jennifer Brown, Noorda College of Osteopathic Medicine

One of the most important parts of the accreditation process falls to the accrediting body designees who are assigned to the program undergoing accreditation or reaccreditation. During an institution's accreditation timeline, any number of persons will be assigned as site inspectors to objectively report their findings to the accrediting body. Understanding what site inspectors are looking for will be helpful in ensuring a smooth process. This chapter will discuss Commission on Osteopathic College Accreditation (COCA) for osteopathic schools and colleges of medicine as well as Liaison Committee on Medical Education (LCME) for allopathic schools and colleges of medicine. Though there will be considerable detail discussed in preparing for these specific accreditation site visits, the approach will be useful to any reader undergoing a site inspection through a different accrediting body.

COCA utilizes both the terms "inspector" and "evaluator" for accreditation assignees, and thus the terms will be used interchangeably throughout the chapter.

PREPARING FOR THE SITE VISIT

Your institution will know who will be on the inspection committee at least two months beforehand. The site visit date will be known two to three months in advance, and your institution's accreditation specialists will submit the necessary required documentation sixty days in advance of the visit. The visit is designed to ensure that your institution is in full compliance with all current accreditation standards and to identify opportunities for improvement over time.

The library benefits significantly from knowing with whom they will be meeting on the committee. If a library representative is not on the preparation team, it is important to be informed of the site inspection process. Some questions that are helpful to ask your institution's planning team:

- Are there any specifics you (the planning team, administration, faculty/staff) need to know about the library as we prepare?
- Are there any specific details the site inspectors are looking for?
- Which designees will be meeting with the library?
- Is there anything the site visit team will be focusing on or interested in when meeting with the library?

Your institution may want to have usage statistics, recent program or instruction data, or even a list of subscribed library resources available in preparation for meetings with the inspection team. The library may be asked to provide a list of employees and their credentials, which may include American Library Association (ALA) accredited program graduates and undergraduate school information. Finally, it may be helpful to have a list of Association of Health Information Professionals (AHIP) credentialed employees who are working at the library.[1] This could be an opportunity to educate site inspectors on this portfolio-based credential that is well known across the health sciences librarianship profession and could also be informative to colleagues who may not know about the credential. Many folks who are aware of the AHIP designation still may not be aware of the four levels that differentiate tenure within the profession.

As a person who will be meeting with evaluator(s) throughout the site visit, you and/or the site inspector assigned to your area have a right of refusal to meet to mitigate any conflicts of interest.

KNOWING WHAT ACCREDITING BODIES ARE LOOKING FOR

Knowledge of what your inspectors are looking for throughout the accreditation timeline will allow for meaningful and structured meetings. Each inspector will be assigned specific areas of the institution to evaluate. For instance, COCA will send your institution a table similar to table 7.1, listing each individual on the team with their credentials along with their expertise and assignments on the committee.

Table 7.1.

Team Members	*Expertise*	*Assignment*
	Administrator and Educator	Team Chair
	Practitioner	Clinical
	Administrator	Student Services
	Academic	Preclinical
	Accreditation Staff	Team Secretary
	Accreditation Staff	Observer

The team composition will be smaller when overseeing an interim or focused review, which can occur between full site visits. Usually, interim or focused teams will be composed of two to three evaluators. This team will be chosen based on the competencies identified for evaluation during the visit.

The lead inspector will oversee the evaluators and will be responsible for compiling the findings from the other evaluators on the team. The areas of focus for a site inspection will fall into the following categories:

- Student Affairs
- Governance and Finance
- Academics and Research
- Clinical

A similar model is used for other accrediting bodies, such as the LCME. Note that the above example references a full COCA site visit. The inspection that your institution may be preparing for could be a focused or interim progress review (the terminologies may vary depending on the accrediting body) and thus may have fewer members on the team.

Libraries will almost certainly fall under the purview of the academics/research evaluator. The accreditation web pages can be full of useful information as you prepare for your site visit. Most prominently, accrediting bodies list the standards used to accredit institutions. Knowing where the library delivers on the relevant standards will be an asset in your preparation.

The following standards can be covered from library services (see table 7.2).

Table 7.2.

COCA Standard	*LCME Standard*
4. Facilities	3. Academic and Learning Environments
6. Curriculum	4. Faculty Preparation, Productivity, Participation, Policies
7. Faculty and Staff	5. Educational Resources and Infrastructure
8. Scholarly Activity	6. Competencies, Curricular Objectives, and Curricular Design
10. Graduate Medical Education	7. Curricular Content
11. Program Assessment and Outcomes	8. Curricular Management, Evaluation, and Enhancement

COCA STANDARD 4: FACILITIES

"A COM [College of Osteopathic Medicine] must have sufficient physical facilities, equipment, and resources for clinical, instructional, research, and technological functions of the COM. These resources must be readily available and accessible across all COM locations to meet its needs, the needs of the students consistent with the approved class size, and to achieve its mission."[2]

Inspectors in this area will be determining if the facilities are adequate for the capacity of the program(s) in question. Are the library physical spaces enough to accommodate the students of a doctor of osteopathic medicine (DO) program? Institutions in candidate status (prior to pre-accreditation) only need to demonstrate the planned facilities and how they fit with the overall mission and vision of the institution.

Standard 4.4, a subsection of Standard 4, delves further with Learning Resources. A list of the library resources may be requested by your administration to determine sufficiency of access. It is recommended to have a copy of this report on hand during your meetings. These library resources may include journals, journal packages, databases, tools, pertinent books, and e-books. Inspectors may wish to know about access restrictions as well. Having a list of seat-limited resources is suggested. Your inspector is trying to understand ease of access for students. If meeting virtually or in person, your evaluator may ask you to demonstrate how to access these resources from the library website.

As of 2022, the table to submit under section 4.4 appears as follows:

Table 7.3.

Resource Type	*# Available*	*Electronic, Paper, Other*	*Specify If Other Was Selected*	*For E-Resources, # of Users Permitted*	*Purpose*
This is where you will list the name of the resource, such as ClinicalKey and DynaMed.	This is the number of licenses available, if the resource has only a finite number of licenses.	What type of resource this would be within the collections. Electronic and paper are the two more common formats in this table.	If choosing Other, specify in this column. This could be other resources that don't fit either category, such as unique and noteworthy items available for checkout within the library's holdings.	For resources that have a seat number, this is the column where that number will be specified. If this is an unrestricted, campus-wide resource, simply mark "Unlimited."	Choose the category that best fits this resource. Many books will fall under "Reference." Textbook collections should be stated as such. Clinical tools, board prep resources, and anatomy should be described accordingly.

If the COM is not standalone—that is, if it is a part of a greater university system—then there is a host of resources that are likely available via the greater campus library system. Students and faculty alike will likely have access to these resources by virtue of being affiliated with the institution. Be sure to consider these resources for inclusion in any relevant reporting to COCA.

LCME Standard 5: Educational Resources and Infrastructure will be comparable for the allopathic medicine accreditation standards. Specifically, 5.8: Library Resources and Staff and 5.11: Study/Lounge/Storage Space/Call Rooms are areas in which you may be able to expound on the adequacy of the library study spaces in relation to the needs of the student population.[3,4]

COCA STANDARD 6: CURRICULUM

Libraries provide perpetual access to resources that are critical for the execution of the curriculum in the modern-day college/school of osteopathic medicine.

Unique to colleges of osteopathic medicine, faculty practitioners in osteopathic manual manipulation (OMM) and osteopathic principles and practice (OPP) will engage in teaching and research. Section 6.6 discusses OPP in specifics. Having a well-equipped library that provides services and resources will be a useful service to a DO practitioner faculty. Osteopathic medicine has many niche resources that are especially valuable for DO faculty. Questions that may be asked in this category include how the library manages library access for part-time table trainers and preceptors.

Standard 6.11 describes comparability across clinical sites. Very few DO degree granting institutions have a hospital attached to the college. This means that it is more likely that students will need to travel to satisfy requirements for their clinical experiences at a variety of clinical sites. Being physically located on the institution's main campus for core rotation experiences is less likely. Wherever the student is located geographically, it is important that they have equal access to resources at each clinical site. There may be questions the site inspector asks about how students can get access to the library when they are away on rotations.

Historically, the requirement was a physical collection at each clinical location. A small, in-print collection would be housed to satisfy this standard. We are lucky this requirement is no longer in place.

LCME Standard 6.3 refers to self-directed and lifelong learning. Specifically, "[Self-directed learning] involves medical students' self-assessment of learning needs; independent identification, analysis, and synthesis of relevant information; appraisal of the credibility of information sources."[4] Librarians who teach evidence-based medicine, critical appraisal, searching the literature, and/or information literacy as part of a curriculum will fall into this category. Depending on how pronounced librarian/librarian faculty involvement is, this could also extend to LCME Standard 7.

COCA STANDARD 7: FACULTY AND STAFF

For schools and colleges in candidate status or undergoing continuing accreditation, the requirement is standard: faculty and staff must be properly qualified to perform in the roles in which they are employed. Librarians fit into this category. Professional librarians on staff who possess an earned MLS from an ALA-accredited program satisfy this requirement for Standard 7. As previously discussed, this could be a great opportunity to provide education on AHIP credentialing.

The conversation may be different depending on the status of librarians at the institution. If librarians are staff, it may be a simpler conversation. If librarians are faculty, be prepared to discuss the library track for faculty development and progression, which should be available as part of rank and promotion information in the faculty handbook.

A sufficiently staffed library is only the first step. Showcasing how the library carries out the greater mission of the college fits well within this standard.

For LCME accreditation, Standard 5.8: Library Resources and Staff is the section where you will be able to elaborate on the credentials of the library team.

COCA STANDARD 8: SCHOLARLY ACTIVITY

Will you be able to articulate the scholarly agenda for your institution? How ambitious is the research mission, and does the library have the resources on hand to carry it out? If not, do you know what is currently missing and when it can be fulfilled? Are you in active discussions with your college's research leaders?

If the school does not have a pronounced focus on research, as is less likely at an allopathic institution than an osteopathic one due to related accreditation standards that vary significantly from COCA to LCME, site inspectors may focus less on the need for research-specific resources. For larger research-based institutions, these questions are more likely. The same can be expected for land-grant, Association of Research Libraries (ARL) members, and flagship institutions.

Inspectors may ask which library faculty or staff members handle research requests for your institution. This could take the form of literature reviews, consultations, and systematic reviews if this amenity is offered through your library. You may also be asked who on your team can specifically support the research agenda. This may include personnel involved in the first question, but also library staff who may have key roles in partnering with the research apparatus of the institution. Staff that handle poster printing, data management, or 3D printing/fabrication labs will all potentially fit into this category.

Finally, COCA Standard 7.3 discusses OMM & OPP research. This standard and your library's role in meeting it will be similar to Standard 6 as it relates to OPP faculty.

For LCME accreditation, Standards 4.2 and 4.5 (Scholarly Activity and Faculty Professional Development, respectively) can allow you to elaborate on scholarly resources for faculty. If your library offers any of the research services discussed above, it will fall under the purview of faculty professional development.

COCA STANDARD 10: GRADUATE MEDICAL EDUCATION (GME)

Graduate Medical Education is another area that utilizes library services at multiple sites, as aspects of your institution's GME program may be geographically diffuse. Many colleges of osteopathic medicine work with a sponsoring institution. These entities may be spread across the state, region, or nation. One such library supports GME efforts in five distinct states where the library provides services. Sponsoring hospitals may have an onsite library but may benefit from the connection to your library and the greater supply of resources and services your library can offer.

Evaluators may ask which GME programs you support. You could be asked about the relationship between the library and the residency programs supported. These questions will be asked for programs that are both nearby and far away and are designed to elicit information regarding equity of service delivery independent of distance from campus.

Pro tip: Determining which resources are currently available at each different clinical site can best illustrate the understanding of the service and resource needs of your affiliates. Knowing which gaps are suitably covered by your library in relation to the learning resource centers at each clinical site will demonstrate an impressive understanding of your institution's GME apparatus. Know your network!

COCA STANDARD 11: PROGRAM ASSESSMENT AND OUTCOMES

This standard focuses on the continuous quality improvement initiatives of the institution. As a part of program assessment, here are a few topics site inspectors may wish to understand in greater detail:

- How do you know how your students are using your library?
- Are you monitoring when patrons are turned away due to seat restrictions?
- What is the library's process of evaluating resources?
- What is your budgeting process like?
- How do you engage in the budgeting process?
- Do you have enough support?

The last question may be infrequently asked in relation to the others. You may be asked to provide examples of evaluation and assessment. If you are already filling out statistics for AAHSL, IPEDS, and any other body that requests an annual usage report, this will provide excellent structure for your responses.

Providing access to library resources is a constantly moving target. Sometimes links go down and proxy stanzas need to be updated. You may wish to provide your team's approach to ensuring continuity of access to resources. Find out ways in which you can demonstrate to the evaluator that regular maintenance and upkeep is being done on the library website and collections.

Finally, this standard is a great way to showcase the library's missional parallels with that of the institution. Telling the site inspector how you and your team are continually improving to meet the growing needs of the program and its patrons is an excellent way to elevate visibility of the library's important role within the institution.

GETTING TO KNOW YOUR SITE INSPECTOR

During the accreditation process, your institution will get a schedule of the upcoming meeting(s) with the site inspectors. At the very least, if your institution has a site inspector meeting with the library, you will have the benefit of knowing who your inspector is beforehand. You may have been provided the entire schedule as well. Either of these scenarios will be excellent opportunities to strengthen the library's role as a critical component of the collective interview process.

Once you have the name of the representative(s) you are scheduled to meet, it is time to research their role and the context from which they operate. Knowing a representative's current title and institution is the most basic context and can be provided by your institution's accreditation specialists or leadership in advance of the visit. Here are a few questions to ask beyond basic demographic information:

- Where else has this person worked?
- What are (if any) their experiences with the library and using library services?
- What courses do they teach? What courses have they taught in the past?
- Have they published research in any discipline-specific journals?
- What were their roles at previous institutions?

Having answers to these questions will allow you to better understand their relationship with the libraries they have interacted with in the past. You may or may not be able to discern comprehensive answers to these questions. As much information as you can ascertain will be helpful in having a productive meeting with them. Do this for each member of the committee with whom you may be meeting.

Visiting the library website(s) from their current and previous institutions will provide you a window to how they currently may be utilizing library resources and services. Some questions to consider:

- If they teach a class, what is the level of cooperation that is visible from the library/school of medicine website? Do they have any course reserves in place? Are course guides for any of the classes that they teach hosted on the library website?
- If they conduct any research, what is the coverage of the discipline they teach on their current institution's website? In what journals have they published? Do they have published books that are available through library holdings?

Once you have a general idea of what interactions your interviewer may have in utilizing library services and resources, it is time to learn how your library presence satisfies these same requirements. For instance, if your interviewer is a published author in a notable biochemistry journal whose title is available at their institution, they may already be looking into whether your library has the same coverage. It would be a smart and proactive move to have this information internalized prior to your meeting. Adding these points within your notes for your meeting(s) will create a structured point of reference from their perspective.

If you are provided a full schedule and list of inspectors, it may be beneficial to do the same for each of the other inspectors. If you believe that any of your colleagues may be discussing any of the points in which the library is involved, as discussed in the previous section, providing them with this information could be helpful.

THE INTERVIEW

There should be no new information on the day of the interview that will surprise the interviewees on the schedule. A visit serves as an affirmation of what has already been submitted to the inspection team. Be prepared to discuss what has been submitted in the latest report. The questions will predominantly relate to what has been submitted. If there is a question that you are surprised by, a simple "To make sure I'm accurate, let me pull up my notes to verify" will allow for some time to collect your thoughts and respond in a prepared manner.

It could be helpful to have an a la carte report of the library section(s) of the submission. This may make things easier. The inspector will likely have a copy of the report and their own notes to refer to during these meetings. Both parties having a copy will allow for precision with the time allotted in the meeting.

Bring additional items that showcase the library in case you satisfy all the interviewer's questions with time to spare in the meeting. If the inspector is open to hearing more, this can be a great time to discuss some of the library's accomplishments over the reporting period that are not covered in the submitted report. However, proceed only if the inspector is open to receiving this information. Read their body language. They have two full days with your institution and have many meetings and duties on this assignment.

Finally, note that your inspector may be on a different schedule. If your institution is on the East Coast and they flew in from the West Coast, there may be a three-hour time difference if they flew in just a night or two before. Be mindful that if your meeting is happening at 10:00 a.m., their internal clock might still be set at 7:00 a.m. Do what you can to be a gracious host.

There may be follow-up after the meeting. Almost always, the follow-up for additional information will only happen if something was not clear in the reports and subsequent meetings. More likely, any follow-up might be based on personal interest and not necessarily related to the inspection.

CONCLUSION

Program accreditation is essential for any medical school to obtain and maintain. It allows programs to accept federal student aid dollars and qualify for regional accreditation application, and instills confidence in the quality of the program to stakeholders. While the accreditation process is lengthy and detail oriented, preparation for a site visit can be relatively painless if you have the right systems and data collection schedules in place. Collecting data and information retroactively for inspection visits that can be as far apart as ten years for COCA and eight years for LCME can be overwhelming and extremely time intensive. The authors recommend that you plan for accreditation-related records to be generated and archived regularly as an ongoing component of your annual academic cycle.

An understanding of the goal of the site visit, individual evaluators, their personal relationship to library services, and your potential interactions with them will help you to be as organized, professional, and prepared as possible. By using the resources and strategies outlined in this chapter, you can make the process smoother and become an expert ambassador for your library not only with accrediting bodies but with all the institution's stakeholders as appropriate.

NOTES

1. Medical Library Association, "MLA AHIP Credentialing: Academy Value to Employers," accessed May 15, 2022, https://www.mlanet.org/page/elevator-speech-for-employers.
2. Commission on Osteopathic College Accreditation, *Accreditation of Colleges of Osteopathic Medicine: COM Continuing Accreditation Standards* (Chicago: Commission on Osteopathic College Accreditation, 2019), 51.
3. Liaison Committee on Medical Education, *Functions and Structure of a Medical School: Standards for Accreditation of Medical Education Programs Leading to the MD Degree* (Washington, DC: Liaison Committee on Medical Education, 2021).
4. Commission on Osteopathic College Accreditation, *Evaluator Manual* (Chicago: American Osteopathic Association, 2017), 25.

BIBLIOGRAPHY

Commission on Osteopathic College Accreditation. *Accreditation of Colleges of Osteopathic Medicine: COM Continuing Accreditation Standards.* Chicago: Commission on Osteopathic College Accreditation, 2019, 51.

———. *Evaluator Manual.* Chicago: American Osteopathic Association, 2017.

Liaison Committee on Medical Education. *Functions and Structure of a Medical School: Standards for Accreditation of Medical Education Programs Leading to the MD Degree*. Washington, DC: Liaison Committee on Medical Education, 2021.

Medical Library Association. "MLA AHIP Credentialing: Academy Value to Employers." Accessed May 15, 2022. https://www.mlanet.org/page/elevator-speech-for-employers.

8

Partners in Accreditation

LIBRARY CASE STUDY AND SUGGESTIONS FOR BEST PRACTICES

Elizabeth G. Hinton, Susan B. Clark, and Mitzi R. Norris, University of Mississippi Medical Center

Libraries are a vital part and partner in accreditation and should embed processes to facilitate both institutional and programmatic accreditations within day-to-day activities and data collection. While not entirely commonplace in the literature, cases of librarians' involvement in accreditation efforts have been documented for many years. Numbers of librarians participate in reaccreditation interviews for specific programs, and several other librarians have used the application of accreditation standards as a reason to embed themselves into the curriculum. Aligning with the standards of the Accreditation Council for Graduate Medical Education (ACGME) standards, a graduate medical education (GME) librarian position was created at the University of South Florida to serve a consortium charged with expanding GME programs in the state of Florida.[1] Dexter and colleagues incorporated Liaison Committee on Medical Education (LCME) and Commission on Osteopathic College Accreditation (COCA) accreditation standards into the creation of several twenty-first-century medical libraries.[2] A nursing librarian at the Hampton University School of Nursing described the experience of helping her institution achieve full accreditation during two separate site visits.[3] In multiple instances, health sciences librarians have leveraged medical education accreditation standards to integrate into the medical school curriculum at their various institutions.[4,5,6]

The Association of College and Research Libraries (ACRL) *Framework for Information Literacy for Higher Education* was originally created as "an education reform movement" meant to give structure to the redesign of information literacy instruction.[7] Several health sciences librarians have connected the framework to programmatic accreditation standards. In 2018, a group of librarians from the Association of Academic Health Sciences Libraries (AAHSL) Competency-Based Medical Education Task Force mapped the framework to the Association of American Medical Colleges (AAMC): Core Entrustable Professional Activities for Entering Residency and the ACGME Common Program Requirements.[8] Brennan and colleagues built upon AAHSL's preliminary work by expanding the mapping of the ACGME Common Program Requirements to the ACRL Framework in 2020.[9] Young and Hinton mapped the framework components to several health sciences program accreditation standards (specifically nursing, dentistry, pharmacy, medicine, occupational therapy, physical therapy, and veterinary medicine) in 2019.[10]

Libraries must report statistics for a variety of reasons; most health sciences librarians are familiar with yearly reports for organizations such as AAHSL. Health sciences libraries can be either stand-alone libraries or a division of the main university library. Regardless, the health sciences library needs to keep distinct statistics to report yearly growth in collections and increased use of services. Benchmarking against peer institutions is not only helpful for accreditation but is a valuable tool for monitoring adequate numbers of staff, services, and collections. While benchmarking is important for the library to tell a story to administration, it is also important in making a case for various institutional, school, and program accreditations. Accrediting agencies ask for both similar and different information in making a case for accreditation. Accrediting agencies may ask specifically for some metrics, or they will expect the institute to demonstrate that the library has an adequate collection, a qualified staff, and suitable services for patrons served. Reporting librarians must read the questions and standards carefully to understand exactly what is being asked and measured and to ensure that all reporting is consistent across all surveys and throughout the accreditation narrative.

A "boilerplate" document can be very useful for keeping up with library statistics for a variety of reasons:

- All information is recorded in one place, thus assuring consistency in reporting.
- Data can be easily updated.
- Not all recorded information will apply to every survey, but parts can be pulled out for various needs.
- New sections can easily be added as the need arises.
- The document is not publicly available, so it is possible to notate when and where various sections were used.
- Statistics for the boilerplate document also correspond to the annual report.

NAME OF LIBRARY

Write statement about history of library, who named for, significant events for library

Mission Statement with date of revision (if any)

Facility

- Basics: location on campus; date of construction; square footage for each floor; square footage for storage and/or archives
- Type of furniture: carrels/tables/chairs (include use if necessary) and number of each
- Special areas (for students or other): group study rooms/collaborative areas/classrooms/lounges and number of each

Access/Hours

- Who has access? Does access vary for specific users?
- Hours: total number; staffed hours; summer/holiday/break hours
- Parking and how to access (badge swipe, etc.)
- List website and how to access e-resources

Services

- Interlibrary loan and potential fees; orientation; printing
- Wi-Fi availability statement
- Other services: EndNote training; systematic reviews; research impact; writing center
- Distance students: services and collection access; photocopy/email/mail services for on-campus materials

Collections keep updated yearly

- Print books/journals
- Electronic books/journals
- Databases
- Major packages

Staff

- Number and qualifications of professional librarians
- Number of staff positions

Links to necessary documents:

- Policies: library/collection development
- Procedures to request new resources

Figure 8.1. Sample Boilerplate Document

Figure 8.1 provides a template for a boilerplate document with suggestions for included statistics. This document should include a statement about the library and its background or history and a current mission statement with date of latest revision. The physical library should be described in detail to include location, date of construction, square footage, type and number of furniture pieces, and any special areas like student lounges or makerspaces. Access and hours should be recorded to describe who, when, and how: *who* has access, *when* they have access, and *how* they access materials, space, and staff. Services will list information about library basics, such as printing and Wi-Fi, and more specific services like classes and research support. Resources for distance students should also be addressed in the services section to demonstrate that library services for those off campus are equal to the services offered to on-campus students. Collections, which should be updated yearly or as needed throughout the year, should be both adequate in number and availability of access and appropriate for the populations served by the institution. The boilerplate document should list numbers of print titles, electronic titles, databases, and any major publisher packages that the library licenses. Staff should be listed by number and qualifications of degreed librarians and number of staff positions. Further, website links to pertinent documents such as the library's policies (access services, collection development, and so on) or other procedures should be listed for easy access.

LIBRARY BACKGROUND

Institutions of higher learning are dynamic organizations. To maintain relevance and meet workforce needs, changes are inevitable. New degree programs are developed, departments merge, and programs are removed from the institution's degree profile. These and other changes affect the operations within the academic unit. However, these changes also affect many administrative functions within the institution.

To mitigate these changes, the University of Mississippi Medical Center (UMMC) established the Potential Academic Change Committee (PAC). PAC was established to bring together individuals whose areas of responsibility could be affected by academic changes; one of the areas affected by academic changes is the Rowland Medical Library (RML). Prior to the establishment of the committee, casual conversations, or internal communications among individuals in affected areas, worked disjointedly to usher in new programs or to implement other academic changes. The committee was established to formalize the communication among affected administrative areas. The original composition of the committee included enrollment management, financial aid, assessment, institutional research, student information system, and accreditation. As the committee established its processes, the need for the involvement of library administration was noted, and this role was added to the membership.

Although the development of new programs rests with faculty, the committee oversees the process to ensure institutional policies and external expectations are met. According to UMMC's website, the charge of the PAC is "to ensure the proper planning and implementation of new academic degree programs, oversee the development of new academic units, and manage modifications to existing academic units or degree programs." The committee directs the schools to ensure compliance with federal financial regulations, governing board guidelines, and institution-wide accreditation standards. The PAC Committee augments the processes within the Office of Enrollment Management (OEM) and with the student information system.[11] The committee meets monthly or as needed, and email is used to communicate immediate changes. PAC has institutionalized and standardized processes: schools and programs consult with PAC as changes are considered. As PAC has become embedded into the academic community, the process has provided efficiencies and allowed for easier implementation of academic changes. The inclusion of PAC in the process has resulted in information about academic changes coming to the forefront earlier and, thus, increasing the efficiency and timeliness of implementing new programs or making other necessary changes.

The designated representative from each area addresses the academic change as the change relates to the area. For example, when a new program such as the doctor of occupational therapy was added, the change triggered notifications to the governing body and institutional and programmatic accreditor. Through representation on PAC, the library was informed about this important program change. Because doctoral programs have research requirements, the library noted the change and reviewed the holdings to determine if new resources were needed for the program. Rowland Medical Library keeps an updated collection development policy that is frequently used when submitting yearly institutional effectiveness reports (IEPs). Specific educational programs are selected for an assessment cycle—the library collection is compared to the current needs of the program—and every attempt is made to improve library resources for the program. Personnel resources are also vitally important: knowledge of potential new programs through membership in PAC gives the library director notice to review liaison assignments. The liaison librarian, along with the director, needs to be aware of any programmatic accreditation requirements that present additional library involvement beyond numbers of holdings. It is possible that the liaison librarian could need additional continuing education opportunities to meet the needs of the new program.

LIBRARY CASE STUDY FOR PROGRAMMATIC ACCREDITATION

With time, many healthcare professions advance the educational level for entry into the profession. This was the case for occupational therapy. In 1999 the programmatic accreditor, Accreditation Council for Occupational Therapy (ACOTE), voted that the professional entry level for occupational therapy programs must be offered at the post-baccalaureate level by January 1, 2007. In April 2019, after an extensive review, ACOTE decided not to require a doctoral point of entry. Instead, the determination was that occupational therapists could enter the profession at the master's or doctorate level.[12] However, the program at UMMC made the long-term decision to move forward with the transition to the doctoral level.

PAC

For the occupational therapy program at UMMC, the process to change from the master's level to a doctoral degree began with a communication from the program director inquiring about how to proceed in September 2015. The PAC chair provided information about institutional expectations and communicated deadlines for submission. Information was submitted to the governing board in March 2016.

GOVERNING BOARD

The Board of Trustees of State Institutions of Higher Learning (IHL Board), an active policymaking governing board that is the legal body with specific authority over the institution, governs UMMC. The IHL Board oversees all public institutions with four-year or higher degrees. Each institution is required to gain approval for new programs or other academic actions, and the IHL Board Office for Academic and Student Support provides guidelines about reporting changes. The institution must demonstrate the new program is within the scope of the institutional mission. Additionally, programs must document adequate faculty, a developed plan of study for students, mechanisms to evaluate, and resources to support the program.

UMMC submitted the required information to the IHL Board proposing the new doctoral-level program in occupational therapy, and the request was approved.

INSTITUTIONAL ACCREDITATION

The Southern Association of Colleges and Schools Commission on Colleges (SACSCOC) is UMMC's institutional accreditor. UMMC provided a prospectus that detailed the proposed program, faculty, faculty qualifications, plan of study, availability of appropriate space and resources, and the projected timeline to implementation. An important section of the prospectus included information about the institution's library resources specific to the program. The library provided a detailed list of appropriate books, journals, and databases that would be available for faculty and students in the program.

PROGRAMMATIC ACCREDITATION

The Accreditation Council for Occupational Therapy Education (ACOTE) is the programmatic accreditor for occupational therapy programs. The organization must grant approval before any new programs can be added. The process for approval includes a self-study. Section A.2.14 in the ACOTE standards addresses "Library, Reference Materials, Instructional Aids, and Technology." Expectations are specified for each level of degree, from associate to doctoral.[13]

EXECUTION

Approval was obtained from the governing board, institutional accreditor, and programmatic accreditor. The program director and faculty began planning the changes, and the school administrators allocated resources for the changes. The new program underwent initial accreditation procedures for the doctoral-level program. The process incorporated a review of the didactic and clinical experience of the students, qualifications of faculty, assessment plan, and appropriateness of resources (including the library) and institutional support.

PULLING IT ALL TOGETHER

As the new doctoral program began, students in the existing program matriculated through the master's degree program. As the last student graduated, the governing board was notified that that program was discontinued. Additionally, ACOTE was notified to discontinue accreditation of the master's degree program as the program transitioned to the new doctoral-level program. The notification to the programmatic accreditor required a notification to the institutional accreditor that there had been a change in accreditation status for a program at UMMC. ACOTE accepted voluntary withdrawal of accreditation of the master's degree program. At the same meeting, the doctor of occupational therapy (OTD) program at UMMC was granted a status of accreditation for a period of seven years.

Information about all degree programs including the OTD program were included in the institutional reaccreditation documents for the institutional accrediting body's ten-year reaffirmation. The program was listed in the sections about programs and faculty. In addition, the accreditor was listed as a programmatic accreditor and the standards were referenced to document a valid program.

STRATEGIES FOR IMPLEMENTATION

The goal of accrediting agencies is to make sure academic programs meet the basic standards of higher education and meet the changing needs of students. While there are certain commonalities within each agency's standards, each agency writes to address the specificity of their respective professions. Becoming familiar with the library's role in the various institutional, school, and program-specific accreditation reporting and staying current on accreditation standards will create the foundation for successful accreditation visits.

A boilerplate document with possible questions and measures that the library can consult when called on to provide documentation or a response can also aid in streamlining the process of new program accreditation and reaccreditation efforts. In the case of the occupational therapy program's degree change from master's to doctoral level, both the library's close relationship and involvement with the Office of Academic Effectiveness, the PAC, and the maintenance of an up-to-date boilerplate document provided efficiency in this part of the accreditation process.

NOTES

1. Laura A. Murray and Candice J. Kunkle, "Defining GME Librarianship: Creating and Developing a New Graduate Medical Education Library Program and Librarian Position," *Medical Reference Services Quarterly* 40, no. 4 (2021): 355–68, https://doi.org/10.1080/02763869.2021.1987773.
2. Nadine Dexter et al., "Building New Twenty-First Century Medical School Libraries from the Ground Up: Challenges, Experiences, and Lessons Learned," *Journal of the Medical Library Association: JMLA* 107, no. 1 (2019): 6–15, https://doi.org/10.5195/jmla.2019.493.
3. Cynthia Burke, "Nursing Accreditation: What's a Librarian Got to Do with It?" *ABNF Journal: Official Journal of the Association of Black Nursing Faculty in Higher Education* 14, no. 2 (2003): 45–46.
4. Claudia Kaufman, Suzy Conway, and Kathy E. Gallagher, "Health Information Resources: Tradition and Innovation in a Medical School Curriculum," *Medical Reference Services Quarterly* 18, no. 1 (1999): 11–23, https://doi.org/10.1300/J115v18n01_02.
5. Diane G. Schwartz et al., "The Health Sciences Librarian in Medical Education: A Vital Pathways Project Task Force," *Journal of the Medical Library Association: JMLA* 97, no. 4 (2009): 280–84, https://doi.org/10.3163/1536-5050.97.4.012.
6. Natalie Tagge, "Leveraging Accreditation to Integrate Sustainable Information Literacy Instruction into the Medical School Curriculum," *Journal of the Medical Library Association: JMLA* 106, no. 3 (2018): 377–82, https://doi.org/10.5195/jmla.2018.276.
7. Association of College and Research Libraries, *Framework for Information Literacy for Higher Education*, accessed February 10, 2022, https://www.ala.org/acrl/sites/ala.org.acrl/files/content/issues/infolit/framework1.pdf.
8. Association of Academic Health Sciences Libraries (AAHSL) Competency-Based Medical Education Task Force, "Health Information Literacies Competencies Map," accessed February 10, 2022, https://www.aahsl.org/assets/docs/Health%20Information%20Literacy%20Competencies%20Map%20%28excel%29.pdf.
9. Emily A. Brennan et al., "Introducing a Health Information Literacy Competencies Map: Connecting the Association of American Medical Colleges Core Entrustable Professional Activities and Accreditation Council for Graduate Medical Education Common Program Requirements to the Association of College & Research Libraries Framework," *Journal of the Medical Library Association: JMLA* 108, no. 3 (2020): 420–27, https://doi.org/10.5195/jmla.2020.645.
10. Lauren M. Young and Elizabeth G. Hinton, eds., *Framing Health Care Instruction: An Information Literacy Handbook for the Health Sciences* (Lanham, MD: Rowman & Littlefield, 2019).
11. University of Mississippi Medical Center Office of Academic Affairs, "Potential Academic Changes," accessed February 10, 2022, https://umc.edu/Office%20of%20Academic%20Affairs/About-Academic-Affairs/Academic%20Effectiveness/Potential%20Academic%20Changes/Potential%20Academic%20Changes.html.

12. American Occupational Therapy Association, Inc., "History of AOTA Accreditation," accessed February 10, 2022, https://www.aota.org/education-careers/accreditation/overview/history.aspx.
13. Accreditation Council for Occupational Therapy Education (ACOTE), "2018 Accreditation Council for Occupational Therapy Education (ACOTE) Standards and Interpretive Guide," accessed February 10, 2022, https://acoteonline.org/wp-content/uploads/2020/10/2018-ACOTE-Standards.pdf.

BIBLIOGRAPHY

Accreditation Council for Occupational Therapy Education (ACOTE). "2018 Accreditation Council for Occupational Therapy Education (ACOTE) Standards and Interpretive Guide." Accessed February 10, 2022. https://acoteonline.org/wp-content/uploads/2020/10/2018-ACOTE-Standards.pdf.

American Occupational Therapy Association, Inc. "History of AOTA Accreditation." Accessed February 10, 2022. https://www.aota.org/education-careers/accreditation/overview/history.aspx.

Association of Academic Health Sciences Libraries (AAHSL) Competency-Based Medical Education Task Force. "Health Information Literacies Competencies Map." Accessed February 10, 2022. https://www.aahsl.org/assets/docs/Health%20Information%20Literacy%20Competencies%20Map%20%28excel%29.pdf.

Association of College and Research Libraries. *Framework for Information Literacy for Higher Education*. Accessed February 10, 2022. https://www.ala.org/acrl/sites/ala.org.acrl/files/content/issues/infolit/framework1.pdf.

Brennan, Emily A., Rikke Sarah Ogawa, Kelly Thormodson, and Megan von Isenburg. "Introducing a Health Information Literacy Competencies Map: Connecting the Association of American Medical Colleges Core Entrustable Professional Activities and Accreditation Council for Graduate Medical Education Common Program Requirements to the Association of College & Research Libraries Framework." *Journal of the Medical Library Association: JMLA* 108, no. 3 (2020): 420–27. https://doi.org/10.5195/jmla.2020.645.

Burke, Cynthia. "Nursing Accreditation: What's a Librarian Got to Do with It?" *ABNF Journal: Official Journal of the Association of Black Nursing Faculty in Higher Education* 14, no. 2 (2003): 45–46.

Dexter, Nadine, Joanne M. Muellenbach, Elizabeth R. Lorbeer, Debra Rand, Matthew E. Wilcox, and Bradley A. Long. "Building New Twenty-First Century Medical School Libraries from the Ground Up: Challenges, Experiences, and Lessons Learned." *Journal of the Medical Library Association: JMLA* 107, no. 1 (2019): 6–15. https://doi.org/10.5195/jmla.2019.493.

Kaufman, Claudia, Suzy Conway, and Kathy E. Gallagher. "Health Information Resources: Tradition and Innovation in a Medical School Curriculum." *Medical Reference Services Quarterly* 18, no. 1 (1999): 11–23. https://doi.org/10.1300/J115v18n01_02.

Murray, Laura A., and Candice J. Kunkle. "Defining GME Librarianship: Creating and Developing a New Graduate Medical Education Library Program and Librarian Position." *Medical Reference Services Quarterly* 40, no. 4 (2021): 355–68. https://doi.org/10.1080/02763869.2021.1987773.

Schwartz, Diane G., Paul M. Blobaum, Jean P. Shipman, Linda Garr Markwell, and Joanne Gard Marshall. "The Health Sciences Librarian in Medical Education: A Vital Pathways Project Task Force," *Journal of the Medical Library Association: JMLA* 97, no. 4 (2009): 280–84. https://doi.org/10.3163/1536-5050.97.4.012.

Tagge, Natalie. "Leveraging Accreditation to Integrate Sustainable Information Literacy Instruction into the Medical School Curriculum." *Journal of the Medical Library Association: JMLA* 106, no. 3 (2018): 377–82. https://doi.org/10.5195/jmla.2018.276.

University of Mississippi Medical Center Office of Academic Affairs. "Potential Academic Changes." Accessed February 10, 2022. https://umc.edu/Office%20of%20Academic%20Affairs/About-Academic-Affairs/Academic%20Effectiveness/Potential%20Academic%20Changes/Potential%20Academic%20Changes.html.

Young, Lauren M., and Elizabeth G. Hinton, eds. *Framing Health Care Instruction: An Information Literacy Handbook for the Health Sciences*. Lanham, MD: Rowman & Littlefield, 2019.

Part Three

Debrief: Action Items for Follow Up

9

Debrief with the Library Team

Rhonda L. Altonen, Touro University

What is debriefing? Debriefing is a structured learning process designed to evolve plans while they're being executed continuously. It originated in the military to learn quickly in rapidly changing situations and address mistakes or changes in the field.[1] Webster's definition includes references to interrogations and law enforcement questioning. Debriefing has been practiced in these contexts to recap and strategize for future events. The second referenced definition states, as a transitive verb, "to carefully review upon completion" and gives an example of using the word in a sentence, a quote from Sean Cantwell in his *Forbes* article, "The best CEOs reach out ahead of board meetings to discuss the upcoming agenda and follow up after to *debrief* to discuss additional insights."[2] The act of debriefing means carefully examining and analyzing upon completion, providing a succinctness to and a summary of a situation. In this chapter we will discuss the debrief, what it is, the research, and its role and purpose in the accreditation cycle.

WHAT IS DEBRIEFING?

Debriefing has long been recognized as playing an essential role in learning when experience alone is considered insufficient to produce understanding. Indeed, debriefing is viewed by some as the "most valuable component . . . in producing gains in knowledge."[3] Without people even realizing it, debriefing is a daily exercise in most professions: business, politics, law enforcement, psychology, healthcare, law, and so on. It is often seen as integral to an organization as members reflect on their learning experiences, track their progress, and gain more understanding. While there is a significant amount of literature on debriefing, especially in recent years, it is mainly found within medicine, nursing, and other health-related practice-based professions.[4] Much of the focus has been on debriefing in simulation exercises in medical and nursing training, which has tended to dominate thinking about what debriefing is and how it should look.[5]

As the accreditation process comes full circle, the reports are submitted, and the experience can now be put behind you. The next accreditation process is years away. Once the accreditation interviews and visit are done, you might think you and your staff can relax; the impulse to get back to your routine of reference, education, circulation, meetings, and assisting patrons is strong. Contrarily, now is the time to take a moment to reflect and consider what you can do to make the process easier, less stressful, more organized for the next accreditation cycle. Details can be easily missed, because not everyone is going to remember everything that happened during the visit and interviews.

Debriefing is built into the accreditation visit. Chapter 1 explains the history of the accreditation system in American higher education, which began in the late 1800s and early 1900s as a way for colleges and universities with high academic standards to distinguish themselves from institutions that claimed to be colleges but had curricula similar to many high schools.[6] There are some clinical agencies that follow the practice of debriefing. The Council on Academic Accreditation (CAA) handbook, and the Middle States Self-Study handbook have built debriefing into the accreditation visit. As part of the CAA Accreditation Quality Management System, at the conclusion of each face-to-face meeting, council members conduct a verbal debriefing in closed session to evaluate the effectiveness of the meeting, including the agenda, materials, resources, and staff involvement. In addition, each CAA member completes a written evaluation, which is submitted anonymously.[7] The Middle States Self-Study manual includes debriefing as part of the agenda for the self-study preparation visit; the team schedules daily meetings to evaluate its progress, adjust assignments, and assess the need for additional information.[8] You may have been a part of the accreditation cycle and process and have a good understanding of the months and years of meetings that are involved. The accreditation cycle involves education, clinical, and hospital providers in continuous improvement and a demonstration that they meet the high standards of quality required to improve student learning. As far back as 1974, the phrase "accreditation cycle" has been used to identify the process of accreditation for higher education institutions.

Keep in mind there are a lot of components to accreditation: an application process and set of threshold criteria by which organizations are eligible to apply for accreditation; a process of self-evaluation; an external evaluation process, including site visits by external accreditors; an appeals process for accreditation determinations; and finally a repeat cycle of self-evaluation and external evaluation.[9] Whether your library played a small or large role in accreditation, the planning and preparation is a time-intensive endeavor. It places the library in the same cycle of continuous quality improvement that the organization faces. Before you know it, the cycle starts all over again. In all the planning and preparation and meetings, was debriefing part of the process? The program accreditation of postsecondary schools or programs takes place on a cycle that may range from every few years to as many as ten years, depending on the accrediting body.[10] We are all part of the process, with debriefing as that point that then connects you to the next point, the final report. You might ask, "Why bother with a debriefing meeting?" With all the meetings, interviews, and tours you are giving during accreditation, you and your staff are continually taking notes, whether mental or written, making observations, and seeing your library and its services in a different light. Taking time at the end of each day during the process and making notes is informal debriefing. Take the next step to create a more formal process for the library staff and even the institution as a whole.

DEBRIEFING AS PART OF THE ACCREDITATION CYCLE

Debriefing is a worthwhile and effective tool to promote quality improvement and improve staff workflow within the department. Many institutions have begun to utilize continuous quality improvement (CQI) as part of their accreditation process. CQI has also been referred to as Total Quality Management, Quality Improvement, Six Sigma, Kaizen, and a variety of other labels. CQI is both a process and a support system that organizations use to identify problems they want to solve, identify strengths that work in their favor, and focus on innovation and growth. The principles for CQI can be found in a variety of forms in healthcare, and have been numbers as few as four and as many as seven. The essential core principles focus on processes, not people. CQI examines the organization's system and its processes to maximize its business operations with the focus on outcomes. CQI is inclusive; teams are drawn from various stakeholders including employees, management, volunteers, board members, and customers. Quality improvement is the responsibility of the whole team, not just management. CQI is empowering; all stakeholders are empowered to identify variations and/or errors as well as opportunities for improvement. Individuals are encouraged to develop and present solutions. Lastly, CQI uses the scientific method, which involves the collection, analysis, monitoring, reviewing, and adjusting to information obtained about processes and systems. It uses the scientific method approach or "trial and error" to measure systems and processes. Teams observe, measure, and then experiment with changing different variables to see which combinations produce the best results.[11] Continuous quality improvement processes should close the feedback loop. The Accreditation Council for Graduate Medical Education's (ACGME) Next Accreditation System (NAS) explicitly adopts CQI principles. The Liaison Committee on Medical Education (LCME), which accredits MD degree programs in the United States and Canada, revised its standards in 2015 to include CQI. In addition, several medical schools have incorporation CQI as part of their accreditation process, going so far as to create CQI accreditation subcommittees. Adding CQI into the accreditation process results in the improvement of results that are then used for program improvement. Improvement of the process is the end goal.

LEARNING THEORY AND DEBRIEFING

Accreditation takes time, and it can be mentally, physically, and emotionally draining. In her blog, *Academic Excellence. Nothing Less*, Dr. Roberta Ross-Fisher posts that "Accreditation Stress" is real.[12] Ross-Fisher has several suggestions that tie right back to using the debriefing to make the process easier. Preparing ahead of time and scheduling the debriefing meetings can be a part of the process. Providing training to faculty and staff, again, would include the training on how to conduct a debriefing, what the goals and expectations are. Delegation can also make the process go more smoothly, having a facilitator to guide the flow of information. That person should also play the primary role in delegating tasks to appropriate personnel. They maintain a schedule to complete tasks on time.

Getting everyone on board for including a debriefing might be a challenge, especially if it is not considered necessary; a short-sighted attitude of "we have been doing it this way, it works, why change?" is often the most used reason. Evidence, mainly from research on health simulations, shows that debriefing promotes a range of skills, knowledge, and personal development and reinforces the need for debriefing. An informal question posted in October 2021 to MEDLIB-L—an email discussion list for medical librarians—asked members if they included a debriefing meeting as part of their accreditation process, specifically for higher education institutions. Only two responses were received, both from hospital librarians, and they referenced debriefings only after clinical simulation sessions. No mention of post-accreditation debriefing meetings was provided. David Kolb is an American educational theorist and one of the forefathers of experiential education philosophy. Kolb believed that to truly learn from experience, there must be time for reflection and review. The reflective observation, abstract conceptualization, and active experimentation elements are most directly connected to debriefing as the time to reflect on an event, examine its meaning through the team's filters, and create a new model that can be applied to future accreditations.[13] Debriefing is a core component of Kolb's experiential learning cycle and is where the bulk of learning takes place. Learning researcher Graham Gibbs discussed structured debriefing to facilitate the reflection involved in Kolb's experiential learning cycle. Taking the time to reflect on and recognize the knowledge, skills, and attitudes used in an experience, learners develop personal awareness and insight. They become aware of their own resources that they can use in future experiences.[14]

Fey equates debriefing as a reflective discussion, "guided by a facilitator that attempts to bridge the gap between experiencing an event and making sense of the event."[15] Reflection enhances learning from experience and expands our knowledge. Promoting the use of reflective practice improves judgment. However, learning from reflection is not automatic and demands active involvement in the relevant experience. Recent work has started to explore the effectiveness of various debriefing strategies/approaches, for example, self- versus facilitator-led debriefing, structured versus unstructured debriefing, single versus co-debriefing and in-person versus tele-debriefing.[16, 17, 18] Interactive debriefing techniques are supported by Kolb's learning theory. Debriefing with a facilitator is considered critical for the process of experiential learning.[19] The facilitator guides the debriefing process to reach established, predefined debriefing objectives. When debriefing is unstructured, unpredictable learning outcomes occur, and it is challenging to ensure that the objectives have been met. In comparison, when a structured debriefing process is established, a safe environment for reflecting and receiving feedback is formed.[16] Cheng defines co-debriefing as more than one facilitator conducting a debriefing session, when these facilitators may be from the same or different departments. Ideally, co-debriefing aims for co-facilitators to work together to manage discussion in a fluid fashion that promotes effective learning.[20] A critical advantage of co-facilitation is the potential for facilitators to complement each other's styles, to provide a larger pool of expertise. However, challenges can arise between co-facilitators that can lead to confusion and discord. Facilitators have differing personal agendas, lack of understanding of the identified objectives, and lack of expertise with the department they are co-debriefing. A debriefing meeting with your team can be seen as an experiential learning scenario/facilitated reflection/reflective discussion that can be a beneficial collaborative endeavor to provide valuable insight as you continue your accreditation cycle.

Is there a debriefing scheduled as part of your accreditation process? If not, start small. Make the debrief meeting part of your department's meetings, and make sure everyone is aware of the debriefing, its goal/purpose, and any expectations you have. Take a further step back and have a "pre-briefing" where all of this can be reviewed. If there is any lack of clarity, the rest of the debriefing will be of little value because you won't know how to measure your results. Start with some general objectives and consider what are you trying to achieve with the debriefing. Consider how the interviews were handled. Did the tours go well? Did everyone know what their roles were? What worked, what didn't, and what can be improved next time? Next, clarify your role in the debriefing meeting. You are there to guide the discussion, participate as a co-learner, and then provide some expectations and the goal for the meeting.

ANATOMY OF A DEBRIEFING MEETING

What does a debriefing look like? A debriefing meeting is more than a casual conversation to discuss what did and didn't go well. Debriefing digs into why things happened and explores implications for the future of that project or plan. Accurate understanding and knowledge are placed ahead of staff egos. Team members participate with a desire to truly understand the root causes of their successes and failures so they know what to repeat and what to change. The conversations may be uncomfortable, but participants realize that the discomfort of getting things out on the table is minimal compared to the pain of making the same mistakes again.

The debriefing meeting(s) should have a goal; these meetings provide a sharing of knowledge, challenges, and feedback. Your library staff becomes a sounding board in a supportive environment to facilitate a better process. Consider what happens if you lose key staff before the next accreditation visit. You might lose any notes or observations they made during the process, especially if they are part of the administrative team and played a key role in the visit. What about when a new person joins the team just before an accreditation visit? Starting a new job has its own stress and learning curve; coming in just before an accreditation visit without preparation might be a breaking point for a new employee.[19] A debriefing allows for better preparation for existing staff and provides new/incoming staff a reference to review. Staff responsible for reporting to their supervisors will have notes to refer with context to their roles and experiences. Note-taking can be challenging, and trying to remember what you meant at the time is confusing. Notes from a debriefing can contain more valuable information; they can incorporate details you might have missed and context from your colleagues as they are experiencing the process from their perspective.

The best time to schedule a debriefing meeting with your staff is while everything is fresh in your collective minds. Notes that you took on the fly might not make sense when you read them after months or even a few years later. Statements made or observations can be lost in translation or through the filter of our thoughts and experiences. What topics can you include in your debriefing agenda? You could all share your thoughts on the process: what worked, what didn't, and what you might change for the next visit. Some additional topics to consider as part of the debriefing could include discussing whether the tours went well. Was the library shown in its best light during the tour, and was it the best time of day? Maybe it was too quiet or too busy; that can make for more stress and be reflected in the report. Another point of discussion is making sure there is enough staff to manage the visit and conduct regular, day-to-day duties. Also, were all the library staff aware of the visit and what the roles and expectations for the day were? If there is an unexpected staff absence, is there a staff person prepared to fill in for that role? If the visit is scheduled during exams, how will that affect the library schedule, and can it be rescheduled, or do you find a workaround? What worked well, and do you want to make sure you include it for the next visit? It's possible that the library space itself won't be included in the tours; instead, there may be meetings with individual staff or departments and accreditation team members as part of the visit. What was the library staff experience and their takeaways from these meetings?

Consider creating a template for your debriefing meetings. Start by using existing meeting outlines, noting what components to keep and identifying what you want your debriefing meeting to look like and include. At a minimum, include agenda items that ask the following questions: What went well, what didn't and why, what should we do differently or similarly next time? According to Doug Sundheim, there are four key steps to an effective debriefing meeting. First, schedule a regular time and place. The key here is to make the debriefing expected, so everyone adopts the same mindset before the activity at the center of the debriefing. When people know they're going to be getting together afterward and can anticipate the general structure of the conversation, they'll begin gathering insights in advance. Eventually, the more you debrief, the more effective and efficient the process will become. Make sure to create a learning environment. Goals and objectives should be made clear, so the team knows the purpose, not one's position on the organizational chart. The leader in the room sets the tone. The expression "leave your ego at the door" applies here. People making themselves vulnerable and admitting to errors gives everyone permission to do the same. Lastly, everyone should consider what was learned. Make sure you capture what was discovered in a usable format for later referencing. At a minimum, this is taking notes and distributing them to the members present.[1]

David Pendleton, professor in leadership at Henley Business School, has developed "Pendleton's Rules." These are rules that help trainers give balanced feedback to trainees.[21] The idea is that, when giving feedback, learners should concentrate on the positive first and then say what they thought could have been done better. Pendleton's Rules are first to clarify any points of information and then ask what was done well and ensure that they identify the strengths of the performance and do not stray into weaknesses. Next, discuss what went well, adding personal observations; if there is a group observing the performance, ask the group what went well; again, keep them to the strengths. Then ask the learner to say what went less well and what they would do differently next time.[22] Finally, discuss what went less well, adding your observations and

DEBRIEF model

Describe events as factually as possible
Evaluate what went well/to change next time
Banish emotions/beliefs/assumptions that cloud judgement and development
Review and analyse in light of previous experience (pattern recognition)
Identify lessons learned
Establish follow up actions
Feedback on actions

Figure 9.1. Allan's DEBRIEF Model
SOURCE: ©HAYLEY ALLAN 2009

recommendations (if there is a group observing the performance, ask the group to add their observations and recommendations).

In her paper, "DEBRIEF: A Reflective Tool for Workplace Learning," Hayley Allan reviews Pendleton's work and takes it a step further by creating the DEBRIEF Model. DEBRIEF is a tool that enables reflection between several people or individuals. It provides a structure for reviewing an event in emotional, cognitive, and practical ways, thus addressing the psychosocial and practical elements of learning. The DEBRIEF model helps learners "take responsibility for their learning, to be autonomous thinkers, develop integrated understandings of concepts, and pose—and seek to answer—important questions."[23] The DEBRIEF model uses the first letters of each word as an outline, as shown in figure 9.1. Allan has created a series of questions asked of the learner that promote the recall and reflection of the events and an evaluation of their role in the events. Reflection often follows the experiential learning cycle of Kolb.

If this is not your first accreditation experience, think back on previous accreditation visits you have participated in, and think about what happens after each meeting. Your mind is full. If you are with a small group, you all might start discussing the event and how you feel. What you thought during the event and asking those with you their thoughts are part of the debriefing. Seeing the experience from other team members' perspectives can enhance your own to a point or observation that you missed during the visit. Try to build in short debriefings throughout the visit if feasible. If that is not possible, provide notebooks for you and your staff and take the time to express your thoughts and feelings about what happened after each event. Using a conversational format will allow staff to synthesize their ideas and motivate your library staff, and they will be more comfortable as this will feel less like an interview. Having a conversation versus an interview is more relaxing, with less stress to provide the "right" answer.

Your role as the facilitator will be to assist the learners, your staff, in examining the event, their thoughts, and even the emotions that occurred during the visit. In their 2013 literature review, Lusk and Fater reviewed debriefing literature in various disciplines, which provided some insight into the structure and process of debriefing. One of these processes was the facilitator's responsibility to provide a safe environment, use active listening techniques, and encourage reflective discussion by everyone.[24] In making it a safe environment, the facilitator engages the learner, creates an inviting learning environment, and establishes psychological safety. Psychological safety is essential to debriefing. Psychological safety is defined as the ability to "behave or perform without fear of negative consequences to self-image, social standing, or career trajectory."[25] For this requirement, learners must be able to express their opinions without fear of personal harm or rejection. If the team is not working together up to expected standards, the facilitator should examine the situation that led to the actions observed. Your library team should be active participants in a confidential debriefing meeting, and the focus is on the accreditation visit outcomes instead of individual criticism. A shared mental model allows both the facilitator and learners to have a mutual understanding of events.

WHAT DEBRIEFING IS NOT

Debriefing is never one-way communication. Use this as an opportunity to "vent" or express your initial feelings and thoughts. You can always go back later and organize them for the debriefing discussion. Keep in mind that you set the tone of the meeting. When you make yourself vulnerable and admit to mistakes, it permits everyone else to follow your lead. The other key aspect of creating a learning environment is not pointing fingers or assigning blame. For example, lack of trust influences personal insecurities, leading to micromanagement. Micromanagement is defined as the ability "to manage with excessive control or attention to details." Micromanagement will most likely deliver poor results, stifle creativity, limit employees' self-worth, and limit productivity. Micromanagement has been proven to be a stressful management style that achieves results only in the short term and can be extremely taxing on both team members and management, which only adds to the stress of the accreditation process. You can avoid micromanaging the debriefing by keeping open lines of communication with your team. A strategy to avoid micromanagement of the debriefing is to set expectations early in the process. Another contributor to micromanagement is a fundamental misunderstanding or miscommunication between the manager and team members. If this breakdown in expectation-setting occurs, it becomes hard for employees to produce work that the manager wants to see, which, in turn, opens the door for micromanagement.

If you can set clear-cut expectations early on when scheduling the debriefing sessions, you will likely see work that aligns with those expectations. It gives your team enough time to assess how they can achieve the goals you have set and eliminates any guesswork on the part of the team that may lead to ill-advised strategy or production. Making sure the team is aware of the expectation of the debriefing in conjunction with your accreditation visit is a great way to avoid any misunderstandings and the previously mentioned finger-pointing. You can create a clear and concise game plan and forge ahead with the accreditation visit.

Lack of communication can also contribute to finger-pointing moments. Communication issues are among the most mentioned concerns when working in a team setting. After every planning meeting, there is a universal desire to "improve communications." The problem is that it is focused on the symptom, not the problem. In almost all cases, if the root cause is revealed as "lack of communication," it results from nonexistent or poorly devised procedures. In other words, staff does not know when they have completed a specific action. They need to follow up with other departments, log the activity, or initiate dissemination of the information to someone. A brief discussion in any planning group about this situation will confirm that written procedures and staff training could rectify the problem. Lines of communication need to be consistent and strong.

The good and bad results should be considered team results, recognizing that everyone had a hand in creating them. Some topics should be included in the debriefing, and some should be excluded. Conflict-based issues shouldn't remain unaddressed at the end of a project, but they also have no place being argued around others on the team. These issues should be handled behind closed doors. It isn't appropriate to discuss publicly who made mistakes because blame isn't constructive, especially in front of others. It can lead to grudges and resentment. Take on concerns forthrightly. Be open to discussion when you see conflict, whether the visit isn't progressing as you'd like or a staff member isn't approaching the debriefing in the way you'd expect. That might mean giving simple feedback, working to develop a staff member's skills, or tackling a serious performance issue or a fundamental problem with fitting the role.

Remember that debrief meetings should be constructive; no personal gripes should be aired. The biggest hurdle to debriefing is merely starting it, especially if you have an organization or even department where this sort of open communication isn't the norm. If that's the case, start small. If you just completed your accreditation or know you will be starting to prepare soon, pick some small projects you might be starting soon and pilot the debriefing as part of the planning meetings. Once you begin adding debriefing to the process, you may quickly realize how natural and intuitive it is for the workflow. Take the time to experiment, talk about what worked and what didn't, and then use that learning to get more thoughtful about your next set of projects. The most effective change processes are usually the simplest.

CONCLUSION

Accreditation is a cycle, and debriefing is one part of that cycle. Debriefing can set the stage by providing the time and space for reflection and focus. Debriefing is extensively used as a teaching and learning strategy across various disciplines. Debriefing can be a powerful tool to assist teams in learning from experience. Using a framework to discuss a gut feeling with a more experienced colleague can lead to unexpected revelations. Debriefing allows learners to feel in control of their work. To learn from the debriefing, individuals on the team must feel safe, and the experience must have a relevant impact. The biggest hurdle to debriefing is merely starting it, especially if you have a culture where this sort of open communication isn't the norm. If that's the case, pick some small projects and a close-knit team to pilot the process. Taking the time to stop and reflect, meet with your department, and review the accreditation process and their thoughts and notes will make the next visit go that much more smoothly and removes much of the stress.[26] Debriefing brings a team together, strengthens relationships, and fosters team learning.

BIBLIOGRAPHY

Allan, Hayley. "DEBRIEF: A Reflective Tool for Workplace Learning." https://www.e-lfh.org.uk/wp-content/uploads/2021/03/DEBRIEF-A-Reflective-Tool-for-Workplacelearning.docx.

Brooks, Jacqueline Grennon, and Martin G. Brooks. *In Search of Understanding: The Case for Constructivist Classrooms*. Upper Saddle River, NJ: Merrill Prentice Hall, 2001.

Brown, Diane K., Ambrose H. Wong, and Rami A. Ahmed. "Evaluation of Simulation Debriefing Methods with Interprofessional Learning." *Journal of Interprofessional Care* 32, no. 6 (2018): 779–81. https://doi.org/10.1080/13561820.2018.1500451.

Cantwell, Sean. "Council Post: You've Raised Capital, Now What? Here Are Four Things to Think About Next." Forbes, 2021. https://www.forbes.com/sites/forbesfinancecouncil/2021/11/01/youve-raised-capital-now-what-here-are-four-things-to-think-about-next/.

Cheng, Adam, Janice Palaganas, Walter Eppich, Jenny Rudolph, Traci Robinson, and Vincent Grant. "Co-Debriefing for Simulation-Based Education: A Primer for Facilitators." *Simulation in Healthcare: Journal of the Society for Simulation in Healthcare* 10, no. 2 (2015): 69–75. https://doi.org/10.1097/SIH.0000000000000077.

"Definition of Debrief." Merriam-Webster.com, 2021. https://www.merriam-webster.com/dictionary/debrief.

Easton, Judith S. *An Overview of U.S. Accreditation*. Washington, DC: Council for Higher Education Accreditation, November 2015. https://www.chea.org/overview-us-accreditation.

Fey, Mary K., Debra Scrandis, Amy Daniels, and Catherine Haut. "Learning through Debriefing: Students' Perspectives." *Clinical Simulation in Nursing* 10, no. 5 (2014): e249–56. https://doi.org/10.1016/j.ecns.2013.12.009.

Harcleroad, Fred F. "Accreditation: History, Process, and Problems." AAHE-ERIC/Higher Education Research Report No. 6, 1980.

Washington, DC: American Association for Higher Education, 1980. https://eric.ed.gov/?id=ED198774.

Institute of Medicine (US) Committee on Assessing the System for Protecting Human Research. *Models of Accreditation. Preserving Public Trust: Accreditation and Human Research Participant Protection Programs.* Washington, DC: National Academies Press, 2001. https://www.ncbi.nlm.nih.gov/books/NBK43596/.

Kolb, David A. *Experiential Learning: Experience as the Source of Learning and Development*. Upper Saddle River, NJ: Pearson FT Press, 2015.

Levett-Jones, Tracy, and Samuel Lapkin. "A Systematic Review of the Effectiveness of Simulation Debriefing in Health Professional Education." *Nurse Education Today* 34, no. 6 (2014): e58–63. https://doi.org/10.1016/j.nedt.2013.09.020.

Lusk, Janet M., and Kerry Fater. "Postsimulation Debriefing to Maximize Clinical Judgment Development." *Nurse Educator* 38, no. 1 (January 2013): 16–19.

McKay, Richard. "Flying the Colors: Coping Successfully with Site Visits from Accrediting Agencies." *Portal: Libraries and the Academy* 4, no. 1 (2004): 145–48. https://doi.org/10.1353/pla.2004.0016.

Middle States Commission on Higher Education. "Middle States Self-Study Guide." Accessed April 5, 2022. https://www.msche.org/accreditation/self-study-guide/.

Oikawa, S., B. Berg, J. Turban, D. Vincent, Y. Mandai, and D Birkmire-Peters. "Self-Debriefing vs. Instructor Debriefing in a Pre-Internship Simulation Curriculum: Night on Call." *Hawai'i Journal of Medicine & Public Health: A Journal of Asia Pacific Medicine & Public Health* 75, no. 5 (2016): 127–32.

Pendleton, David. "Pendleton's Rules." GP-Training.Net. Accessed April 13, 2022. https://www.gp-training.net/feedback/pendletons-rules-feedback/.

Reed, Shelly J. "Measuring Learning and Engagement during Debriefing: A New Instrument." *Clinical Simulation in Nursing* 46 (2020): 15–21.

Reierson, Inger Åse, Thor Arne Haukedal, Hanne Hedeman, and Ida Torunn Bjørk. "Structured Debriefing: What Difference Does It Make?" *Nurse Education in Practice* 25 (2017): 104–10. https://doi.org/10.1016/j.nepr.2017.04.013.

Ross-Fisher, Roberta. "Accreditation Stress: It's Real." *Academic Excellence. Nothing Less* (blog), 2021. https://robertarossfisher.com/2021/02/22/accreditation-stress-its-real-and-you-need-to-prepare-for-it/.

Shinnick, Mary Ann, Mary Woo, Tamara B. Horwich, and Randolph Steadman. "Debriefing: The Most Important Component in Simulation?" Clinical Simulation in Nursing 7, no. 3 (2011): e105–11. https://doi.org/10.1016/j.ecns.2010.11.005.

Stansfield, R. B., Tsveti Markova, and Richard Baker. "Integration of Continuous Quality Improvement Methods into Annual Program and Institutional Evaluation." *Journal of Graduate Medical Education* 11, no. 5 (2019): 585–91. https://doi.org/10.4300/JGME-D-19-00145.1.

Sundheim, Doug. "Debriefing: A Simple Tool to Help Your Team Tackle Tough Problems." *Harvard Business Review*, 2015. https://hbr.org/2015/07/debriefing-a-simple-tool-to-help-your-team-tackle-tough-problems.

Winchester-Seeto, Theresa, and Anna D. Rowe. "Who Is Holding the Mirror? Debriefing and Reflection in Work-Integrated Learning." *International Journal of Work-Integrated Learning* 20, no. 4 (2019): 335–49.

NOTES

1. Doug Sundheim, "Debriefing: A Simple Tool to Help Your Team Tackle Tough Problems," *Harvard Business Review*, 2015, https://hbr.org/2015/07/debriefing-a-simple-tool-to-help-your-team-tackle-tough-problems.
2. Sean Cantwell, "Council Post: You've Raised Capital, Now What? Here Are Four Things to Think About Next," *Forbes*, 2021, https://www.forbes.com/sites/forbesfinancecouncil/2021/11/01/youve-raised-capital-now-what-here-are-four-things-to-think-about-next/.
3. Mary Ann Shinnick et al., "Debriefing: The Most Important Component in Simulation?" *Clinical Simulation in Nursing* 7, no. 3 (2011): e105–11, https://doi.org/10.1016/j.ecns.2010.11.005.
4. Theresa Winchester-Seeto and Anna D. Rowe. "Who Is Holding the Mirror? Debriefing and Reflection in Work-Integrated Learning," *International Journal of Work-Integrated Learning* 20, no. 4 (2019): 335–49.
5. Tracy Levett-Jones and Samuel Lapkin, "A Systematic Review of the Effectiveness of Simulation Debriefing in Health Professional Education," *Nurse Education Today* 34, no. 6 (2014): e58–63, https://doi.org/10.1016/j.nedt.2013.09.020.
6. Fred F. Harcleroad, "Accreditation: History, Process, and Problems." AAHE-ERIC/Higher Education Research Report No. 6, 1980 (Washington, DC: American Association for Higher Education, 1980), https://eric.ed.gov/?id=ED198774.
7. Council on Academic Accreditation in Audiology and Speech-Language Pathology, *Standards for Accreditation of Graduate Education Programs in Audiology and*

Speech-Language Pathology (March 2022), https://caa.asha.org/SysSiteAssets/files/accreditation-handbook.pdf.
8. Middle States Commission on Higher Education, "Middle States Self-Study Guide," accessed April 5, 2022, https://www.msche.org/accreditation/self-study-guide/.
9. Institute of Medicine (US) Committee on Assessing the System for Protecting Human Research, *Models of Accreditation, Preserving Public Trust: Accreditation and Human Research Participant Protection Programs* (Washington, DC: National Academies Press), 2001, https://www.ncbi.nlm.nih.gov/books/NBK43596/.
10. Judith S. Easton, *An Overview of U.S. Accreditation* (Washington, DC: Council for Higher Education Accreditation, November 2015), https://www.chea.org/overview-us-accreditation.
11. R B. Stansfield, Tsveti Markova, and Richard Baker, "Integration of Continuous Quality Improvement Methods Into Annual Program and Institutional Evaluation," *Journal of Graduate Medical Education* 11, no. 5 (2019): 585–91, https://doi.org/10.4300/JGME-D-19-00145.1.
12. Roberta Ross-Fisher, "Accreditation Stress: It's Real," *Academic Excellence. Nothing Less* (blog), 2021, https://robertarossfisher.com/2021/02/22/accreditation-stress-its-real-and-you-need-to-prepare-for-it/.
13. Mary K. Fey et al., "Learning through Debriefing: Students' Perspectives," *Clinical Simulation in Nursing* 10, no. 5 (2014): e249–56, https://doi.org/10.1016/j.ecns.2013.12.009.
14. Shelly J. Reed, "Measuring Learning and Engagement during Debriefing: A New Instrument," *Clinical Simulation in Nursing* 46 (2020): 15–21.
15. Fey et al., "Learning through Debriefing."
16. Inger Åse Reierson et al., "Structured Debriefing: What Difference Does It Make?" *Nurse Education in Practice* 25 (2017): 104–10, https://doi.org/10.1016/j.nepr.2017.04.013.
17. Reierson et al., "Structured Debriefing."
18. Diane K. Brown, Ambrose H. Wong, and Rami A. Ahmed, "Evaluation of Simulation Debriefing Methods with Interprofessional Learning," *Journal of Interprofessional Care* 32, no. 6 (2018): 779–81, https://doi.org/10.1080/13561820.2018.1500451.
19. David A. Kolb, *Experiential Learning: Experience as the Source of Learning and Development* (Upper Saddle River, NJ: Pearson FT Press, 2015).
20. Adam Cheng et al., "Co-Debriefing for Simulation-Based Education: A Primer for Facilitators," *Simulation in Healthcare: Journal of the Society for Simulation in Healthcare* 10, no. 2 (2015): 69–75, https://doi.org/10.1097/SIH.0000000000000077.
21. Richard McKay, "Flying the Colors: Coping Successfully with Site Visits from Accrediting Agencies," *Portal: Libraries and the Academy* 4, no. 1 (2004): 145–48, https://doi.org/10.1353/pla.2004.0016.
22. David Pendleton, "Pendleton's Rules," GP-Training.Net, accessed April 13, 2022, https://www.gp-training.net/feedback/pendletons-rules-feedback/.

23. Hayley Allan, "DEBRIEF: A Reflective Tool for Workplace Learning, "https://www.e-lfh.org.uk/wp-content/uploads/2021/03/DEBRIEF-A-Reflective-Tool-for-Workplacelearning.docx.
24. Janet M. Lusk and Kerry Fater, "Postsimulation Debriefing to Maximize Clinical Judgment Development," *Nurse Educator* 38, no. 1 (January 2013): 16–19.
25. Reed, "Measuring Learning and Engagement."
26. Sundheim, "Debriefing."

10

The Postmortem

HANDLING ACCREDITATION SUCCESS AND FAILURE

Joanne M. Muellenbach, California Health Sciences University

For any activity as critical as preparing for the accreditation of a medical or health sciences program, you should conduct a postmortem review. The postmortem is the phase within a project that analyzes the process's strengths and weaknesses. It provides a unique opportunity for the accreditation team to pause and reflect on the sequence of events, including what went well and where there is room for improvement. The goal of a project postmortem is to gain insight into any circumstances that may result in noncompliance with the accreditation standards and use the findings to improve your process. The information gained through a review of your project's shortcomings can help avoid such mistakes in the future. Concerns about identifying project failures may create a natural disincentive within an institution to conduct a postmortem.[1] It can also cause anxiety for the individuals preparing to participate in this event. However, the accreditation postmortem will help you learn from past successes and failures and further your goals in supporting the university's mission, key initiatives, and outcomes. Therefore, you should be proactive in becoming involved in the accreditation process, ensure a postmortem review process is in place, and share how the results can benefit future accreditation cycles. This chapter will highlight my health sciences accreditation experiences from the perspective of a library administrator, the postmortem review process and how it helped us handle success and failure, and lessons from which you can benefit in the future.

THE JCAH EXPERIENCE

My experience with the accreditation process began in the mid-1980s when I accepted my first full-time professional position as the lead medical librarian at Madison General Hospital in Madison, Wisconsin. The vice president for medical affairs, to whom I reported, provided me with an overview of the Joint Commission on Accreditation of Hospitals (JCAH) process and the opportunity to participate in their upcoming site visits. Given my lack of familiarity with the accreditation process, I called on hospital librarians with whom I collaborated as a member of the Wisconsin Health Sciences Library Association. These colleagues provided suggestions and best practices in preparing for JCAH accreditation site visits. A common theme shared was that the JCAH library standards lacked detail, and efforts to provide librarians with further guidance on their interpretation were progressing slowly. In 1980, Topper and colleagues published a guide for librarians on the JCAH's two library standards, which stated that the library must be well organized and have available written policies and procedures.[2] While further details followed each standard, the mix of specific and vague statements was confusing. Topper's guide was helpful in that it provided interpretations for compliance in staffing, resources, collaboration with hospital administration and other departments, assessments and surveys, up-to-date documentation, and the development of policies and procedures. During our accreditation site visit, the JCAH visitor inspected our library space. The site visitor browsed our print collections and inquired about the availability of specific textbooks, such as Harrison's and a book the visitor, a medical doctor, fondly referred to as the "Green" book, a pediatrics text by Dr. Thomas Green. The JCAH visitor also asked about our staffing, hours, and security, all in less than thirty minutes!

Librarians fulfill many critical roles in today's hospitals, help to maintain the institution's competitive edge, and overall, provide an excellent return on investment.[3] In 2005, following reports of hospital librarians losing jobs and library closings, *Vital Pathways: The Hospital Libraries Project* was established. The Medical Library Association (MLA) president, M. J. Tooey, made it one of her priorities to understand the issues more clearly.[4] Tooey created a steering committee, conducted a survey, and presented a final report to the MLA board of directors, which resulted in the development of a vital pathways symposium to share the project work and ensure the ongoing viability of this segment of medical librarianship. The final symposium paper reported on the plans for repeating the landmark study, "The Impact of the Hospital Library on Clinical Decision Making: The Rochester Study." Marshall's study proved that demonstrating our value can inspire others to achieve similar results.[5] Librarians could also contribute to the accreditation process through ongoing evaluation of their services and demonstrating our impact on the institution's quality culture.[6] In a study by Carpenter, a library collections audit conducted in preparation for a

National League for Nursing accreditation visit resulted in their nursing faculty having an enhanced understanding of their resources and services.[7]

During my years at Madison General Hospital, neither the JCAH nor the hospital administration provided me with any specific feedback regarding our level of library services, positive or negative. The library followed the JCAH's two library standards by being well organized and providing written policies and procedures. The library also gathered and reported annual user satisfaction data and used it to plan future services. In those days and up until 2004, medical libraries had print copies of *Index Medicus*—a comprehensive bibliographic index of MEDLINE articles—and we searched MEDLINE on behalf of our library users. We also provided current awareness services, document delivery, and reference assistance. While we did not receive any direct feedback from the JCAH, the vice president for medical affairs and other hospital leaders showed their appreciation for the library through positive annual reviews and ongoing support. This positive feedback inspired us to continue to provide a high-quality library service and demonstrate our worth. Consumer health information was readily available, and patients were requesting *patient-level* information. We applied for funding through our hospital foundation to develop consumer health information services. We also identified the need to upgrade our audio-visual technology and received funding to purchase new equipment from the same foundation. Later on, the library received a grant to establish a hospital archive and participate in events to celebrate our institution's history.

Reflecting on the library's JCAH experience, our postmortem review consisted of sharing our accreditation experiences with hospital personnel and library colleagues and using the feedback to make positive changes. Overall, I had much to celebrate, but one event triggered a significant change in my career. As a result of our hospital's merger with another hospital, a library colleague became the chief librarian. I used this experience to advance my skills and become professionally active locally and regionally. Ultimately, I accepted an information services librarian/outreach coordinator position at an academic health sciences center library in the western United States, which opened another exciting chapter in my life.

LCME AND CACMS ACCREDITATION

My introduction to the academic health sciences accreditation process began in 2002 when I accepted the position of director, Health Information Resource Centre (HIRC) at the Northern Ontario School of Medicine (NOSM). NOSM, the seventeenth medical school in Canada and the first to be created in more than thirty years, was affiliated with two major universities—Lakehead University in Thunder Bay and Laurentian University in Sudbury. NOSM developed as a strategy to improve physician recruitment and retention in northern Ontario, a vast region of approximately one million people, in an area the size of France, and serving Aboriginal and Francophone populations. The geography and long, cold winters were isolating and made recruiting health professionals difficult. NOSM entered its first class of fifty-six students in fall 2005. During the first two years, the students were distributed between the two main campuses, a distance of 1,200 kilometers. During their third year, students relocated to rural and remote clinical learning sites throughout the north.

As a new medical school library director in Ontario, one of my first responsibilities was to become familiar with the Liaison Committee on Medical Education (LCME) standards for accreditation of medical education programs.[8] The LCME Standard V: Educational Resources (ER) included facilities, finance, information resources, and library resources. The ER-11 standard stated, "The medical school must have access to well-maintained library and information facilities, sufficient in size, breadth of holdings, and information technology to support its education and other missions." ER-12 stated, "The library and information services staff must be responsive to the needs of the faculty, residents, and students at the medical school." Given Standard V's broad focus, NOSM leadership asked the library, information technology, and facilities departments to produce a combined self-study document to show how we met the standard. NOSM was also required to submit documents similar to those needed for the LCME to the Committee on Accreditation of Canadian Medical Schools (CACMS).[9]

The joint accreditation process between Canada and the United States dates back to the 1910 Flexner Report and sets standards for the 134 US medical schools and the 17 in Canada.[10] However, it was the United States that initially set the 131 standards concerning institutions, curriculum, medical student experience, faculty, resources, and procedures. In 2014, Canadian medical schools received the right to set their educational standards and policies, and Canadian accreditors can now review reports, deliberate, and make decisions about Canadian schools. The LCME will then decide whether to accept the decision. If it doesn't, the case goes to a joint committee comprised of the Canadian and US committees and the chair-elect of the US organization, and its decision is final. Most importantly, the CACMS can integrate social accountability standards related to a school's mission to train future physicians and respond to their community's needs, such as those in Aboriginal or Francophone populations. The CACMS can also expand committee participation from students, the public, and experts outside of medical education.

Health sciences libraries were transitioning from print to electronic books, journals, and databases during this period. Accreditors were interested in the library's process for making collection development decisions, whether we had sufficient budget dollars, and how we ensured that faculty, residents, and students had 24/7 remote access. The HIRC was fortunate to be a member of the Consortium of Ontario Academic Health Libraries and participate in electronic resource consortia licensing. Other CACMS and LCME questions for the library focused on our library hours, building security, committee memberships, integration of information literacy and evidence-based medicine (EBM) within the curriculum, and support for our remote users.

The accreditation postmortem review consisted of a team debrief meeting. NOSM leaders shared the accreditation site visit report, invited comments or questions, and allowed us to express our feelings. NOSM also encouraged employees to provide feedback anonymously. The HIRC had submitted a thorough self-study report, and there were no issues that arose at the post-mortem. At that time, most self-study reports provided by medical libraries across the United States and Canada did not result in any "severe action decisions." A study by Hunt and colleagues found that from 1996 to 2000, there were eight citations related to ER-11, and from 2006 to 2009, there was just one citation.[11] For example, in 2013, the CACMS/LCME placed the College of Medicine at the University of Saskatchewan on "Accreditation with Probation." Inadequate study space at their satellite campus in Regina was among the ten issues cited by the CACMS/LCME. Overall, health sciences libraries have successfully interpreted and provided evidence of their compliance with the standards. The HIRC was fortunate to have a sufficient budget to purchase collections, hire personnel, and provide a modern, functional library space. A possible shortcoming for NOSM overall was the high rate of senior administration turnover. A study by Barzansky and colleagues found that senior management turnover was a growing trend across the United States and Canada,[12] and it was no different for NOMS. It was also difficult to find sufficient volunteer faculty to meet the needs of NOSM's distributed medical school curriculum. What felt like a library failure was related to the technological infrastructure of the time and the challenges in providing remote access to library resources. The internet could be unreliable in the faraway northern communities and blocked by hospitals that utilized secure firewalls. As a new medical library director working in a remote community, such challenges were not unusual. I learned the importance of pausing, regrouping, and considering alternative plans to move forward through it all.

Alexander Graham Bell stated, "When one door closes, another opens." In 2008, I became the founding library director for The Commonwealth Medical College (TCMC), a private, not-for-profit, independent medical college with a distributive education model and regional campuses in Scranton, Wilkes-Barre, and Williamsport, Pennsylvania.[13] In 2017, TCMC integrated with Geisinger, a healthcare delivery system, which provided robust clinical learning venues, access to over 1,600 clinical educators to serve as faculty, and exposure to cutting-edge research and clinical innovation in such areas as data science, genomics, informatics, and precision health.[14] I worked remotely from my home in Canada for the first few months, to prepare for TCMC's accreditation site visit, scheduled in July, shortly after my arrival. In October, thanks to the strong leadership of the founding dean and senior leadership, TCMC received provisional LCME accreditation and was given the green light to actively recruit its charter class of fifty MD students and thirty master of biomedical sciences students for fall 2009.

I received a warm welcome from local and regional consortia colleagues. Through my Association of Academic Health Sciences Libraries (AAHSL) membership, I met other directors of new "born digital" libraries—libraries that focused on building digital collections rather than those in traditional print format. We collaborated and shared stories about our accreditation successes and failures. Through our efforts, in June 2012, we received AAHSL support to hold a New Academic Health Sciences Library symposium hosted by the University of Central Florida. With attendees from eighteen new, twenty-first-century medical schools, the symposium featured a keynote presentation by Dr. Robert Sabalis, PhD, assistant LCME secretary and director. Other highlights included panel presentations on budgeting and developing a successful opening-day collection, integration of medical informatics within the curriculum, space planning, and staffing needs. Due to the success of this event, and in light of the growing number of new allopathic and osteopathic medical schools receiving initial accreditation at this time, AAHSL created the New & Developing Academic Health Sciences Libraries Committee, charged with providing networking opportunities for new medical school library directors, training and development, and a feedback mechanism between this committee and other relevant AAHSL committees.[15]

As a participant in the LCME accreditation site visits, I was continuously impressed by the extent to which our senior leaders prepared. The library was responsible for meeting the standards within the self-study that focused on library resources and services. So, the LCME meetings were excellent opportunities to showcase the library's accomplishments, including its effective use of technology, talent for getting to the essence of the users' needs, and deep understanding of library resources for locating evidence-based knowledge.[16] The site visit schedules were prepared and distributed well in advance, complete with photos and brief biographies of the visiting team. At TCMC, we conducted mock site visits, and used the feedback to adjust our processes, responses, and timelines. The LCME accreditation postmortem process consisted of team debrief meetings so that the founding dean and other project leaders could share feedback from the exit interview, their reflections, and their satisfaction with the overall process. The postmortem debriefs allowed TCMC leaders to uncover and analyze any positive or negative findings and make recommendations for changes in the future. As a result of the LCME accreditation postmortem, the importance of the library's contribution to student success became evident.

Through my years of networking with "born digital" library directors for new allopathic and osteopathic medical schools, I have been impressed with the diverse range of roles that my colleagues were taking on. The bottom line is to enhance your library's contribution to student success. You need to review your institution's mission and critical initiatives, identify areas where you can help, embrace change, and reinvent yourself. While at TCMC, I served as coleader of a biomedical informatics thread woven throughout the curriculum. The library team developed online, asynchronous information literacy sessions integrated within a first-year medical school course. In addition, as a member of the Middle Atlantic Region (MCR) of the Network of the National Library of Medicine (NNLM), the library received a Technology Improvement Express award for $10,000 to integrate library resources, technology, and point of care.[17] The library purchased ten tablets for second-year medical students to enable convenient access to the library's clinical and health information resources while in hospitals, physician offices, and clinics to further patient education and support their learning and research. The library also received Outreach to Consumers and Outreach to Health Professionals awards, for a total of $30,000, to enhance access to mental health information for consumers and health professionals. These awards came at a critical period when suicide rates were on the rise across the country. The awards allowed us to collaborate with the Lackawanna County Library System on train-the-trainer events, purchase and provide access to mental health books and media, and promote these resources to consumers and health professionals. As a result, the NNLM Award helped to destigmatize suicide and mental illness and better prepare academic and public librarians on the front lines.

In 2016, I accepted an offer to become the Founding Health Sciences Library director for the new school of medicine (SOM) at the University of Nevada Las Vegas (UNLV). My immediate task was to ensure that we met the revised LCME Standard 5.8: Library Resources/Staff of the DCI.[18] There was not a moment to lose, given that the SOM charter class of fifty medical students was arriving in July 2017. I soon hired new health sciences librarians and professional and classified support staff, and the librarians served on SOM committees and obtained faculty input on collections, services, and space. We collaborated with faculty to design curriculum-integrated instructional sessions focused on information literacy and EBM to further student success.[19] The Health Sciences Library director and dean, UNLV Libraries, participated in the LCME accreditation site visits and the postmortem process. At the postmortem debrief meetings, we shared what went well along with areas for improvement, and we celebrated our successes. Among the library's achievements was developing a series of articles on building "born digital" medical libraries from the ground up, published in the MLA News.[20] The LCME accreditation process also leveraged the library's ability to integrate information literacy and EBM into the medical school curriculum and enhance our students' ability to become lifelong learners. In addition, faculty reported improvements in the range of information sources that first-year medical students cited as part of their curriculum coursework. A case study reported a similar experience in how a medical school and health sciences library leveraged accreditation to develop a sustainable and efficient flipped classroom model for teaching information literacy skills to first-year medical students.[21] An example of an issue that felt like a failure was the slow process for the UNLV SOM to obtain funding for a new medical school building, including a learning resource center/library space. There were several years of back-and-forth between donors and the Nevada System of Higher Education, most notably when a $14 million pledge was withdrawn because then UNLV president Len Jessup left his role. In the end, an organization of philanthropists formed the Nevada Health and Bioscience Corporation (NHBC) and combined their funding and a $25 million contribution from the state. On October 29, 2020, the NHBC broke ground on the UNLV School of Medicine's first permanent structure and the 135,000-square-foot building in Las Vegas's medical district is slated for completion in summer 2022. In the meantime, the UNLV School of Medicine Library and InfoCommons spaces were professionally designed and met the aesthetic and functional expectations of medical students, faculty, and staff, including modern décor, furnishings, equipment, and state-of-the-art technologies. While the space is sufficient for the current class size, the new medical education building will offer the capacity for double, or even triple, the number of students. Staffing two library spaces in separate buildings across the medical district campus could also be challenging, especially when you factor in the extreme Las Vegas heat during the summer months.

THE COCA EXPERIENCE

I was introduced to the accreditation process for colleges of osteopathic medicine (COM) when I joined Touro University Nevada (TUN) as the Director, Jay Sexter Library, in 2018. TUN is a non-profit university focused on positively impacting its community in healthcare and education. The American Osteopathic Association (AOA) Commission on Osteopathic College Accreditation (COCA) "Standard 4.4: Learning Resources" is specific to libraries. It states that a COM must ensure access to learning resources to support its mission. In support of this Standard, libraries are required to submit Table 4.4 to describe the COM's learning resources, including the learning resources of all campuses and affiliated teaching sites to ensure the delivery of the curriculum. To this end, libraries should continuously survey their users' satisfaction levels. In addition, participating in the AAHSL Annual Statistics surveys can help us make a case for new or continuing library resources and services.

As the library director for a relatively young, twenty-first-century medical school library, I was interested in learning about the library's user needs. The library team conducted formal and informal surveys and analyzed the results. Using the results, a case was made for additional funds to create two new librarian positions, renovate the library furnishings, and enhance the library's collections. Another accomplishment evolved from a directive by Touro senior leadership, in anticipation of a new single accreditation system for allopathic and osteopathic medical programs, to enhance the Touro College and University Systems' (TCUS) research footprint. The library team took this opportunity to collaborate with other TCUS libraries and establish a research development webinar series. This series of thirty-minute, research-focused workshops led by librarians from five Touro institutions demonstrated the library's support for faculty and student teaching and research and resulted in excellent publicity. The success of this research series led to a library collaboration with the School of Nursing to become a Joanna Briggs Institute Affiliated Group and provide tools and training in support of systematic reviews.

During my time at TUN, I participated in program accreditation reviews for the college of osteopathic medicine and the school of nursing. The postmortem review processes consisted of debrief meetings for providing direct feedback and making suggestions for changes. At the COCA accreditation site visit debrief, TUN's efforts to enhance its research footprint were lauded, and the library was acknowledged as a vital partner in these efforts. Another success for the library was taking the lead on an NNLM Pacific Southwest Region Express Outreach award for $12,000 that focused on using virtual reality and 3D technologies to expand the health professionals' pipeline in southern Nevada. In addition, for its fifteenth anniversary, the library sought ways to capture TUN's history by taking some initial steps to develop an archive. A task force was formed, comprised of the library and executive leaders, to host and record a panel event with some of the university's founding faculty, staff, and administration. This event served to share and preserve TUN's history of its early days.[22] A possible shortcoming for the library was budget limitations for further development of the library's space. The current library space, consisting of individual carrels, group seating, and lounge furnishing, did not provide room for expansion, nor did it provide adequate office, collaboration, and consultation space. The library space constraints impacted the librarians' ability to meet with students and faculty for systematic review consults or to showcase our virtual reality and 3D technologies.

THE ACPE AND COCA EXPERIENCE

I served as the director of Library and Learning Resources at the California Health Sciences University (CHSU) from 2015 to 2016. Then, in 2019, I was fortunate to have the opportunity to return to CHSU, serve as the director of the Health Sciences Library, and build a brand-new health sciences library from the ground up. Founded in 2012 and envisioned by the Assemi family, CHSU launched its doctor of pharmacy (PharmD) program in 2014. Then, against the backdrop of COVID-19, CHSU enrolled its charter class of doctor of osteopathy (DO) students in 2020. The college of osteopathic medicine (COM) program incorporates a nutrition teaching kitchen, a medical Spanish class, an outpatient and inpatient simulation center, and holographic anatomy, along with active, team-based learning curriculum delivery. As CHSU evolves in its current and new program developments, it will further its mission to address the need for more healthcare providers to care for our ever-growing community, including underserved and rural populations.

One of my first tasks as the library director was to schedule meetings with CHSU administration and department heads to learn more about their areas of responsibility, key initiatives, and accreditation requirements. I also wanted to let them know how the library could collaborate and provide support. For example, as a part of the materials submitted for the Accreditation Council for Pharmacy Education (ACPE) and COCA site visits, the library showcased its efforts to integrate information literacy and EBM within the curricula. We also highlighted our Personal Librarian Program, which provides a concierge-like service to our groups of first-year medical students as they embark on research projects. We act as the single point of contact and provide a full range of research-related services.

In 2020, I initiated a study that involved the collection of data on services and staff practices in academic health sciences libraries serving the college of osteopathic medicine programs. The study data helped to justify the hiring of two new health sciences librarians in preparation for our charter class of medical students.[23] This study also helped raise the library's profile throughout the university and justify the need for sufficient budget dollars for new print and online collections and state-of-the-art learning space, furnishings, and equipment. In advance of our ACPE and COCA site visits, the library created a library and learning resources master list, providing information about and links to the library's print and electronic texts, journals, databases, multimedia, software, and other tools. We also included details regarding the learning resources available through the CHSU Simulation Center, the Office of Academic Affairs and Assessment, and the Office of Student Affairs.

The ACPE and COCA accreditation postmortem processes consisted of online meetings so that our COM and COP program deans could share highlights of the site visit teams' feedback and the next steps in the accreditation processes. We also had the opportunity to comment, ask questions, and receive answers. During the COVID-19 pandemic, the ACPE and COCA site visits were virtual, but despite that, the library team's experiences were positive. For example, the library team met with the COCA site visitor, answered their questions, and had the opportunity to share additional examples of the library's accomplishments, such as the launch of *Scholarly Snippets*, a research development webinar series presented in collaboration with librarians from six other COM institutions across the country in support of faculty, staff, students, and other librarians. The bimonthly webinar topics are recorded and made available on our YouTube channel. We also highlighted our leadership in the development of a CHSU institutional repository for showcasing and preserving the research and scholarship of the CHSU community. Yet another activity through which we contributed to CHSU's success was the receipt of a $20,000 NNLM Express Outreach award in support of a health careers boot camp series to increase the health professions pipeline in California's Central Valley. In addition, we highlighted the library's role in developing a CHSU records management program. Under the leadership of CHSU's president, this program ensures that the university administration, faculty, staff, and students work effectively, reduce costs, maximize space, and comply with all accreditations and licensure and legal requirements. In summary, as librarians, you need to continually align yourself with and promote yourself to your institution or organization as a whole. You must share your skills and talents with others, and while it may mean getting out of your comfort zone, the rewards will be worth it.

As a health sciences librarian involved in the accreditation process and the postmortem reviews, you can play a significant part in the future success of these processes. Participating in the postmortem process design ensures that you will incorporate meaningful learning activities that can inform best practices for future accreditation cycles. You must continually demonstrate your vital role and align yourself with your organization's mission, key initiatives, and outcomes. By promoting yourself, your expertise, and your services, you will continue to be a vital part of your organization. As Maya Angelou stated, "You may encounter many defeats, but you must not be defeated."

LESSONS FROM MY FATHER

In closing, I would like to share a personal story about my father's life and how he inspired me, as a first-generation college student, to be confident, try new things, and not be afraid to fail. Born in 1928 to a single mom who worked at various times as a nanny, beautician, seamstress, and button store owner, my father, having helped his mom with several big sewing orders, found that he had an aptitude for the work. Dad used his talent for sewing while serving in the US Army by sewing buttons on his comrades' uniforms when needed. While stationed in Atlanta, he met his future wife, my mom. My dad worked six days a week and twelve hours per day. His idea of spending time with his six children was to put us to work at the tender age of eight! In addition to Muellenbach Fashions, my father operated Betty Andre's Beauty Salon and the Betty Sullivan Modeling School. Besides sewing and helping out in the salon, Dad loved putting on fashion shows, and we think he thought his kids could entertain his audiences like the von Trapps in *The Sound of Music*. My brother Michael played the organ, and my sisters, any adventurous friends, and I would sing and model during the shows. He thought that we were adorable. At the age of fifty, Dad had the extraordinary experience of being the best man at the marriage of his mother and birth father. My sisters and I served as bridesmaids, wearing original gowns designed by my father. As mentioned earlier, my grandmother worked hard all her life to raise her son independently. At sixty-four, Dad survived gallstone-associated, acute pancreatitis and lived for another sixteen years. My father had a plaque by Sydney Smith displayed above the entrance to his bridal salon's design and sewing area that stated, "A great deal of talent is lost in the world for want of a little courage. Every day sends to their graves obscure men whom timidity prevented them from making a first effort, who, if they could have been induced to begin, would in all probability have gone great lengths in the career of fame. The fact is that to do anything in the world worth doing, we must not stand back shivering and thinking of the cold and danger but jump in and scramble through as well as we can." This plaque could serve as a lesson for us all on how to best handle success and failure.

NOTES

1. B. Collier, T. DeMarco, and P. Fearey, "A Defined Process for Project Post Mortem Review," *IEEE Software* 13, no. 4 (1996): 65–72, https://doi.org/10.1109/52.526833.
2. J. M. Topper et al., "JCAH Accreditation and the Hospital Library: A Guide for Librarians," *Bulletin of the Medical Library Association* 68, no. 2 (1980): 212–19.
3. R. Holst et al., "Vital Pathways for Hospital Librarians: Present and Future Roles," *Journal of the Medical Library Association* 97, no. 4 (2009): 285–92, https://doi.org/10.3163/1536-5050.97.4.013.
4. M. J. Tooey, "A Pathway for Hospital Librarians: Why Is It Vital?" *Journal of the Medical Library Association* 97, no. 4 (2009): 268–72, https://doi.org/10.3163/1536-5050.97.4.010.
5. J. G. Marshall, "The Impact of the Hospital Library on Clinical Decision Making: The Rochester Study," *Bulletin of the Medical Library Association* 80, no. 2 (1992): 169–78.
6. R. F. Dudden, "The Necessity of Measurement," *Medical Reference Services Quarterly* 27, no. 3 (2008): 323–38.
7. K. H. Carpenter, "Evaluating Library Resources for Accreditation: Results of a Study," *Bulletin of the Medical Library Association* 80, no. 2 (1992): 131–39.
8. LCME: Liaison Committee on Medical Education, accessed December 5, 2021, https://lcme.org/.
9. CACMS Secretariat, *Accreditation Documents*, accessed April 8, 2022, https://cacms-cafmc.ca/accreditation-documents.
10. B. Sibbald, "Made-in-Canada Accreditation Coming for Medical Schools," *Canadian Medical Association Journal* 186, no. 2 (2014): E83, https://doi.org/10.1503/cmaj.109-4692.
11. D. Hunt et al., "The Unintended Consequences of Clarity: Reviewing the Actions of the Liaison Committee on Medical Education before and after the Reformatting of Accreditation Standards," *Academic Medicine* 87, no. 5 (2012): 560–66, https://doi.org/10.1097/ACM.0b013e31824d4b7c.
12. B. Barzansky and S. I. Etzel, "Educational Programs in US Medical Schools, 2003-2004." *JAMA* 292, no. 9 (2004): 1025–31, https://doi.org/10.1001/jama.292.9.1025.
13. R. Smego et al., "Anatomy of a New U.S. Medical School: The Commonwealth Medical College," *Academic Medicine* 85, no. 5 (2010): 881–88.
14. A. K. DiMattia et al., "A Snapshot of Medical Student Education in the United States and Canada: Reports from 145 Schools," *Academic Medicine* 95, no. 9 (2020): S426–30.
15. Committees, Task Forces & Representatives—AAHSL, accessed April 9, 2022, https://www.aahsl.org/committees.
16. B. S. Shearer, A. Seymour, and C. Capitani, "Bringing the Best of Medical Librarianship to the Patient Team," *Journal of the Medical Library Association* 90, no. 1 (2002): 22–31.

17. J. M. Muellenbach, "Enhanced Access to Mental Health Information—A Multi-Type Library Collaboration," *Journal of Consumer Health on the Internet* 18, no. 4 (2014): 401–8.
18. N. Dexter et al., "Building New Twenty-First Century Medical School Libraries from the Ground Up: Challenges, Experiences, and Lessons Learned," *Journal of the Medical Library Association* 107, no. 1 (2019): 6–15, https://doi.org/10.5195/jmla.2019.493.
19. J. M. Muellenbach et al., "Integrating Information Literacy and Evidence-Based Medicine Content within a New School of Medicine Curriculum: Process and Outcome," *Medical Reference Services Quarterly* 37, no. 2 (2018): 198–206, https://doi.org/10.1080/02763869.2018.1439225.
20. J. Muellenbach, D. Rand, and B. Long, "Budgeting for an Opening Day Collection in 'Born Digital' Libraries," *MLA News*, January 2016, 22.
21. N. Tagge, "Leveraging Accreditation to Integrate Sustainable Information Literacy Instruction into the Medical School Curriculum," *Journal of the Medical Library Association* 106, no. 3 (2018): 377–82.
22. F. Mazzia and M. De Armond, "Causality Dilemma: Creating a Twenty-First Century University Archive," *Journal of the Medical Library Association* 109, no. 1 (2021): 137–40, https://doi.org/10.5195/jmla.2021.1056.
23. J. M. Muellenbach et al., "Services and Staffing Practices in Academic Health Sciences Libraries Serving College of Osteopathic Medicine Programs: A Mixed Methods Study," *Journal of the Medical Library Association* 108, no. 3 (2020): 408–19.

BIBLIOGRAPHY

Barzansky, B., and S. I. Etzel. "Educational Programs in US Medical Schools, 2003–2004." *JAMA* 292, no. 9 (2004): 1025–31. https://doi.org/10.1001/jama.292.9.1025.

CACMS Secretariat. *Accreditation Documents*. Accessed April 8, 2022. https://cacms-cafmc.ca/accreditation-documents.

Carpenter, K. H. "Evaluating Library Resources for Accreditation: Results of a Study." *Bulletin of the Medical Library Association* 80, no. 2 (1992): 131–39.

Collier, B., T. DeMarco, and P. Fearey. "A Defined Process for Project Post Mortem Review." *IEEE Software* 13, no. 4 (1996): 65–72. https://doi.org/10.1109/52.526833.

Committees, Task Forces & Representatives—AAHSL. Accessed April 9, 2022. https://www.aahsl.org/committees.

Dexter, N., J. M. Muellenbach, E. R. Lorbeer, D. Rand, M. E. Wilcox, and B. A. Long. "Building New Twenty-First Century Medical School Libraries from the Ground Up: Challenges, Experiences, and Lessons Learned." *Journal of the Medical Library Association* 107, no. 1 (2019): 6–15. https://doi.org/10.5195/jmla.2019.493.

DiMattia, A. K., J. A. Arnott, S. Lobo, and W. B. Jeffries. "A Snapshot of Medical Student Education in the United States and Canada: Reports from 145 Schools." *Academic Medicine* 95, no. 9 (2020): S426–30.

Dudden, R. F. "The Necessity of Measurement." *Medical Reference Services Quarterly* 27, no. 3 (2008): 323–38.

Holst, R., C. J. Funk, H. S. Adams, M. Bandy, C. M. Boss, B. Hill, C. B. Joseph, and R. K. Lett. "Vital Pathways for Hospital Librarians: Present and Future Roles." *Journal of the Medical Library Association* 97, no. 4 (2009): 285-92. https://doi.org/10.3163/1536-5050.97.4.013.

Hunt, D., M. Migdal, R. Eaglen, B. Barzansky, and R. Sabasis. "The Unintended Consequences of Clarity: Reviewing the Actions of the Liaison Committee on Medical Education before and after the Reformatting of Accreditation Standards." *Academic Medicine* 87, no. 5 (2012): 560–66. https://doi.org/10.1097/ACM.0b013e31824d4b7c.

LCME: Liaison Committee on Medical Education. Accessed December 5, 2021. https://lcme.org/.

Marshall, J. G. "The Impact of the Hospital Library on Clinical Decision Making: The Rochester Study." *Bulletin of the Medical Library Association* 80, no. 2 (1992): 169–78.

Mazzia, F., and M. De Armond. "Casualty Dilemma: Creating a Twenty-First Century University Archive." *Journal of the Medical Library Association* 109, no. 1 (2021): 137–40. https://doi.org/10.5195/jmla.2021.1056.

Muellenbach, J. M. "Enhanced Access to Mental Health Information—A Multi-Type Library Collaboration." *Journal of Consumer Health on the Internet* 18, no. 4 (2014): 401–8.

Muellenbach, J. M., W. C. Duncan, C. Vanier, L. A. Ennis, and A. Yang. "Services and Staffing Practices in Academic Health Sciences Libraries Serving College of Osteopathic Medicine Programs: A Mixed Methods Study." *Journal of the Medical Library Association* 108, no. 3 (2020): 408–19.

Muellenbach, J. M., K. M. Houk, D. Thimons, and B. Rodriguez. "Integrating Information Literacy and Evidence-Based Medicine Content within a New School of Medicine Curriculum: Process and Outcome." *Medical Reference Services Quarterly* 37, no. 2 (2018): 198–206. https://doi.org/10.1080/02763869.2018.1439225.

Muellenbach, J., D. Rand, and B. Long. "Budgeting for an Opening Day Collection in 'Born Digital' Libraries." *MLA News*, January 2016, 22.

Shearer, B. S., A. Seymour, and C. Capitani. "Bringing the Best of Medical Librarianship to the Patient Team." *Journal of the Medical Library Association* 90, no. 1 (2002): 22–31.

Sibbald, B. "Made-in-Canada Accreditation Coming for Medical Schools." *Canadian Medical Association Journal* 186, no. 2 (2014): E83. https://doi.org/10.1503/cmaj.109-4692.

Smego, R., R. D'Alessandri, B. Linger, V. Hunt, and J. Ryan. "Anatomy of a New U.S. Medical School: The Commonwealth Medical College." *Academic Medicine* 85, no. 5 (2010): 881–88.

Tagge, N. "Leveraging Accreditation to Integrate Sustainable Information Literacy Instruction into the Medical School Curriculum." *Journal of the Medical Library Association* 106, no. 3 (2018): 377–82.

Tooey, M. J. "A Pathway for Hospital Librarians: Why Is It Vital?" *Journal of the Medical Library Association* 97, no. 4 (2009): 268–72. https://doi.org/10.3163/1536-5050.97.4.010.

Topper, J. M. , J. Bradley, R. F. Dudden, B. A. Epstein, J. A. Lambremont, and T. R. Putney. "JCAH Accreditation and the Hospital Library: A Guide for Librarians." *Bulletin of the Medical Library Association* 68, no. 2 (1980): 212–19.

11

Staying in the Conversation

STRATEGIES FOR CONTINUED PARTNERSHIP

Michele L. Whitehead, University of North Texas Health Science Center

As you have learned throughout this text, libraries are critically important in the successful application and receipt of initial accreditation for a new school, college, or degree offering. The required resources, access, space, and education are clearly articulated in some accreditation processes, while others have been interpreted aided by expert librarians who curate resource lists and design best practices based on what is expected of the academic unit or entire institution. Libraries are uniquely positioned to lead in some cases and support in others to ensure that accreditation requirements are initially met, but the real challenge in the journey may begin years down the road after a school or program is more established. Maintaining a partnership with programs, departments, or schools as well as the institutional accreditation and assessment teams is essential and requires the same time, attention, communication, and care long-term interpersonal relationships do to be beneficial to all involved.

Much of the value of the degree conferred to graduates lies in the recognition it carries because of accreditation. Beyond the "street cred" reputation value of being listed among the top-performing, well-known programs in public health or physician assistant studies, for example, in health sciences clinical, biomedical, and public health education, the core competencies found within requirements for accreditation also support the transition from classroom to clinic or professional practice. It is no coincidence that certain expectations exist for medical schools that graduate physicians entering residencies and that accreditation of residency programs carry forward essential knowledge, skills, competencies, and learning conditions that must be provided for new physicians to be successful. Residents entering graduate medical education (GME) from programs that neglected any components of these undergraduate medical education requirements or did not review them early in residency may already be at an early career disadvantage in comparison to their peers.[1] GME accreditation is the continuation of this accountability for educators, even when the teaching is taking place in healthcare practice settings.

The University of North Texas Health Science Center's (HSC's) Gibson D. Lewis Library serves as the setting for the case study described in this chapter of how to ensure the library team is not only included long-term in accreditation discussions but can serve as true, active partners. Arguably, one of the most important best practices a health sciences university can follow for its students is to maintain accreditation in its various programs and schools. This accreditation goes beyond the regional and national higher education institutional-level accrediting bodies to program-specific accreditation that directly impacts the recipient's competitive advantage. National ranking in board exam or certification test scores, postgraduate employment, and other success measures are important but are all arguably impacted by maintaining accreditation.

There is also the importance of health sciences and hospital library professionals' understanding of the scope and progression of biomedical science, clinical, and public health education. For degree-granting institutions that prepare the next generations of information professionals, programs with specific health sciences tracks or specializations can be key in establishing the foundations of this knowledge, but information science programs should include curricula that emphasize how librarians and other information professionals can play a role in their future employer's successes related to accreditation and that it will be an expectation. Even for campuses or schools that do not offer the full range of learning opportunities described in this chapter, or for those that may offer other degree programs, including dental or nursing schools, librarians working to maintain their own growth path and network within the specific disciplines they serve can often find applicable examples to study those that cross disciplinary boundaries. This case study provides a framework of broad, generalizable approaches or strategies for that reason, rather than a specific prescription to follow.

BACKGROUND

In terms of institutional age in comparison nationally to institutions of higher education and some health science centers, HSC is a relatively young campus. The institution began as the Texas College of Osteopathic Medicine (TCOM) and was established with the first class entering in 1970. In addition to TCOM, HSC offers graduate degrees (master's and/or doctorate level) in biomedical sciences, public health, physical therapy, physician assistant studies, and pharmacy. HSC also oversees a postdoctoral residency program for medical school graduates, with residency sites located in facilities throughout the state of Texas, including numerous hospitals in Fort Worth. Gibson D. Lewis Health Science Library (Lewis Library) supports all these users.

HSC is a part of the University of North Texas System (UNTS), but operations and resources of the library are separate from the other campuses, which include a law school and undergraduate programs in Dallas, Texas, and the flagship campus in Denton, Texas. Each unique campus in UNTS also works with other area universities and community colleges in numerous collaborations. One of the most successful on the HSC campus involves interprofessional education bringing together multidisciplinary students for activities designed to enhance each participant's ability to work on teams with a variety of other practitioners where each member provides expertise and perspective.

Lewis Library has been involved with initial and ongoing accreditation for all HSC schools and programs, and the author personally has participated in these processes for more than a decade. During that time, the department of physical therapy in the school of health professions and the HSC college of pharmacy both received provisional and full accreditation, so for the library, the successful launch of these programs has now shifted emphasis to the maintenance of the longer term with an eye on future renewals. This means that consideration for resources that were needed, for example, is now woven into the practices of collection development for those disciplines. The responsibility for knowing the most current information about those programs falls largely on both library administrators and librarians serving as departmental or programmatic liaisons. The programmatic expansion and recruitment of leading teaching faculty and researchers require frequent discussion and updates to resources, educational offerings, and services.

HSC as a case study does offer an enhanced, multisite setting because Lewis Library employees currently also lead library operations for the county hospital through an innovative service agreement with JPS Health Network. The team serves the county's safety net main hospital campus as well as practitioners in more than twenty-five network clinics located throughout Tarrant County. As mentioned previously, Lewis Library at HSC has long served HSC residency programs, but this role in a hospital setting has enhanced the understanding of and participation in the maintenance of accreditation requirements beyond the educational institutional level to the teaching hospital setting.

In working closely with the division of academic affairs, the library participates in the preservation of hospital-level accreditation with the Joint Commission. As an agency, the Joint Commission encourages hospitals to consider the value of this accreditation over the long term because of the significance this well-known accrediting body has as an indicator of quality care, especially for patients in their search for and selection of providers.[2]

HSC library team members working in roles at JPS Health Network often come from academic health sciences library backgrounds or have pursued a health sciences specialization track in graduate school, but not always. Librarians in the hospital setting perform clinical rounds and research for patient care questions in addition to the teaching, scholarship, and networking responsibilities that HSC's academic librarians have. There is a high level of expertise, training, ongoing continuing education, and expectations library administrators set for this team in not only understanding the general practice of long-term involvement in hospital accreditation but also displaying proficiency in medical terminology, practice processes, and the best ways to sustain participation in the GME process.

STRATEGIES FOR CONTINUED PARTNERSHIP

While there are numerous ways libraries attempt to stay involved in accreditation processes with academic departments or medical education divisions, such as by assigning subject specialists or liaison librarians to reach out to those departments regularly, assisting with accreditation can be one of the most important parts of a health sciences specialization. If the library was actively included in the earliest discussions of the formation of schools or programs and involved in the initial accreditation efforts, then a transition can organically begin to maintain involvement over the longer term. If a library was not included or late to enter these discussions, all is not lost. Often the library's position in the reporting structure of the institution or system may play a role in the information sharing, and understanding the significance of this organizational positioning introduces new avenues for entering the conversation.

At HSC, the library's leader, with the title of vice provost for scholarly information resources and university librarian, reports directly to the provost and executive vice president of the university. This organizational positioning regularly provides library administration with valuable information through participation in meetings where many programmatic changes are discussed and solidified by leaders of all colleges and schools the library serves. For those health sciences libraries where leaders report elsewhere, through deans of medical schools or larger university library deans, there are still similar strategies that may be generalizable, but it could be a benefit for library leaders to communicate the value of having a seat at the administrative table that provides the most contact with all programs. In hospital libraries, library leaders having a seat at the academic affairs or GME leadership table is a way to accomplish this.

One suggestion for library leaders in universities where this type of reporting structure is not currently the organizational operational design would be to research other peer institutions, find a model that might lead to enhanced inclusion and communication, and propose this shift in reporting. For the librarians and staff on the team, any elevation of the library's leadership can also pave the way for a tremendous ripple effect and subsequently elevate those tasked with the day-to-day operations at the same time. The true benefit of library leadership involvement at the highest level as possible in the institutional hierarchy related to accreditation is that the library is included in discussions where anticipated issues originate and is able to offer services to assist where appropriate.

In the following sections, the author will address eight distinct strategies and areas of focus to build or rebuild, maintain, and successfully stay involved in accreditation on campus. While these learned experiences are reflected and drawn from lived experience at HSC, the use of this model to validate these strategies will come from consideration and action of those reading this chapter. Arguably, the strategies suggested here are simple, and there are additional strategies that may perform better in other settings. However, the following eight strategies have resulted in sustained involvement of Lewis Library in accreditation processes on the HSC campus over many years and are a place to begin (see figure 11.1).

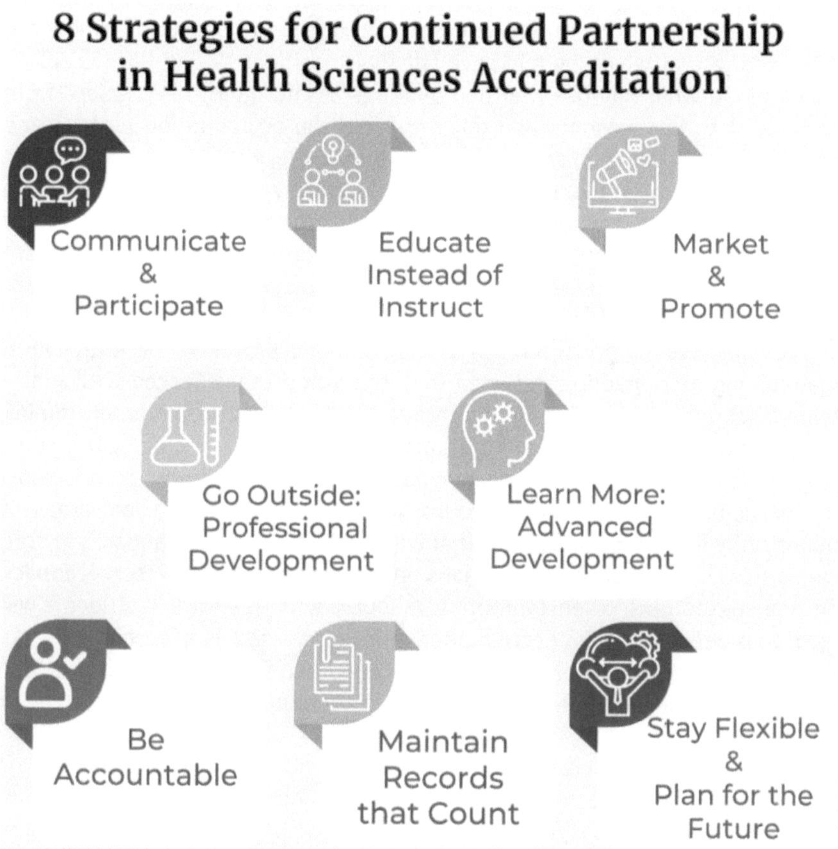
8 Strategies for Continued Partnership in Health Sciences Accreditation
Communicate & Participate
Educate Instead of Instruct
Market & Promote
Go Outside: Professional Development
Learn More: Advanced Development
Be Accountable
Maintain Records that Count
Stay Flexible & Plan for the Future

Figure 11.1. Image by Michele Whitehead

STRATEGY 1: COMMUNICATE AND PARTICIPATE

One of the key ingredients in all successful relationships over the long term is communication and continued investment or involvement. This can present a challenge in the college and university setting and in hospitals for a variety of reasons. For example, staff members on both the accreditation and assessment teams for the institution, the individual academic departments, or the library do experience employee turnover, reductions in funding, and the effects of leadership transition at the highest levels. In recent years, employees nearing retirement have opted for an earlier transition, leaving their roles vacant or strained with interim leadership. With unanticipated departures, one issue arises when these result in losing not only information about the status of work in progress in meeting standards for accreditation but also these employees, especially if long-term, taking a lot of relevant institutional memory with them.

The final strategy covered in this chapter will go into greater detail on succession planning for this very reason, but it is important to note how the increased rate at which people have left their positions during the COVID-19 pandemic in what has been termed by some as the "great resignation" from early 2021 to the present has likely impacted the accreditation process and communication between stakeholders.[3] On a smaller campus or in a practice setting with fewer employees, this may be less likely to happen where people have worked closely with members outside of their departments and want closure to their work, but it is important to anticipate that some may not want recognition, and it can leave vacancies where employees who remain lack closure or proper handoff.

On the HSC campus, several strategies have proven to be effective in maintaining a connection between the library and those tasked with maintaining accreditation requirements through curricular design or programming during any transitions. When librarians can find a seat on curriculum committees or at the very least gain an invitation to observe these working groups, the participation in the course approval process often can reveal areas of opportunity for curricular support that will meet one or more standards or core elements. This also provides librarians an immediate space to insert feedback or offer suggestions, when appropriate, about resources and skills students will need to meet or maintain accreditation standards. There is a learning process in these communications, but librarians can get more familiar with the best ways to communicate and participate by simply being present and listening in these groups.

One way to stay visible and involved for inclusion in departmental or programmatic updates related to institutional accreditation is to also stay involved in other areas of assessment, including the collection, dissemination, and analysis of student satisfaction surveys, facilitation of focus groups, the performance of needs assessments, and through student services partnerships. Library leaders and team members can lead even informally in spaces that require assessment of academic and nonacademic programming by serving on internal councils or committees. In reviewing a program's recruitment and admissions, curriculum, or retention strategies from start to finish and by being involved in the delivery of feedback for suggested improvements, library team members may also learn that by providing input into degree/program-level planning, their understanding for missing support services or unmet needs increases.

Directly related to accreditation and because of the continued library presence related to the collection and analysis of student satisfaction measures, library administrators at HSC were positioned and prepared to serve on the advisory committee for the quality enhancement plan (QEP) required by the Southern Association of Colleges and Schools Commission on Colleges (SACS COC), which operates on a five-year cycle. Library team members have also been included in opportunities to develop programming and education sessions for the QEP.

For example, in the current HSC QEP, Be|Well, Lewis Library's classes and events can be tailored to include topics ranging from organizing digital life to revision of the Paws at Lewis Library certified therapy animal program that began in 2013. These offerings are tied to well-being and student wellness, so it is not unusual to find libraries in the health sciences willing and working to actively participate in this key part of accreditation. The main objective of a QEP cycle is to improve some facet of campus life either in learning outcomes or the overall environment that leads to greater execution of the institution's mission.[4] Library involvement is vital in this process, from research support on the selected objectives to the actual deployment of expertise and programming.

STRATEGY 2: EDUCATE INSTEAD OF INSTRUCT

Academic libraries in higher education have typically always placed emphasis on instruction and teaching as it relates to information fluency and literacy. Librarians in the health sciences should continually attempt to work with faculty to integrate bioinformatics and literacy lessons and practices into the curriculum. At the undergraduate academic level, librarians often lead for-credit, one-hour courses in the identification of different types of sources of information, appraisal of those sources, and strategies in searching. This "Libraries 101" style course is considered the bare minimum for undergraduate degree-seeking students to be thoughtful searchers and consumers of information. But it is typically offered early in their experience, so this basic instruction can present as a vague recollection when reaching graduate school in the health sciences.

The Association of College and Research Libraries' (ACRL's) *Framework for Information Literacy in Higher Education* also provides additional guidance in the essential information literacy knowledge and skills all students should possess after pursuing coursework in a higher education setting. This framework replaced the earlier *Information Literacy Competency Standards* by allowing library educators to shift their focus from following rigid standards to ensuring students were achieving competency in key areas needed to be fluent information seekers and users.[5]

In graduate academic health sciences libraries, research instruction generally includes the emphasis on specific biomedical tools and databases and the importance of evidence in patient care processes. These classes, workshops, or in-curriculum sessions highlight specific issues with scientific inquiry ranging from plagiarism or copyright violations to research integrity issues. The recency of information and its timely distribution become particularly significant considerations in the health sciences, as does the opportunity for the results of publicly funded research to get back into the hands of the public and planning for long-term solutions to the management of health and medical data. Patient privacy, data visualization and management, copyright, systematic review, and professional personas are among popular topics that many libraries offer through education sessions and workshops.

HSC librarians are staff appointments with no faculty status attached at present. For librarian positions that do not earn or have the option to earn faculty status or participate in the pursuit of tenure, several questions arise. Do library administrators focus on filling those positions with trained educators who understand the science of teaching over direct experience in the health sciences? Is there a difference in the expertise of someone teaching in the health sciences library setting who does not have an education or science background? If an adjunct appointment is offered by an academic department, are librarians able to accept outside of their traditional role? Will faculty and students in clinical programs or public health take the teaching of a librarian seriously and integrate librarians into the curriculum as intended without faculty status? How do librarians highlight their expertise in pedagogy/andragogy in addition to their resource and research competence with those audiences?

One shift on the HSC campus that made a significant difference in the inclusion of library instructors as professional educators was the transition in the instructional unit of the library to a method of operating that mirrors that of an education unit or division. This group now functions with similar approaches to academic units where professional practice communities of teachers work collaboratively in course development and a peer-review process exists for courses developed by education librarians. Library educators are recruited and hired for the academic campus for their expertise in pedagogy/andragogy and curriculum design. Library educators are hired in the hospital setting with the added emphasis on experience in the health sciences.

For accreditation purposes, the real benefit to this shift to operations beyond the more traditional instruction/liaison model to function more like education or academic departments is found in the structure it provides. Librarians at HSC are now tasked with creating and maintaining lesson plans, a catalog of courses, putting their courses through a review and approval process in some cases for new course development, and most importantly a mapping of accreditation standards the course content meets in the applicable programs. Courses are no longer developed as just a quick tutorial on how to use a single resource approach, although the tools and resources librarians build do allow the curriculum to be segmented when needed. Quick guides, research guides, videos, and other tools have been invaluable in transitioning to this higher-level preparation, and educator librarians building these courses are required to immerse in the best ways to deliver material and assess student learning. The resources are now incorporated into a skills topic or competency-based course

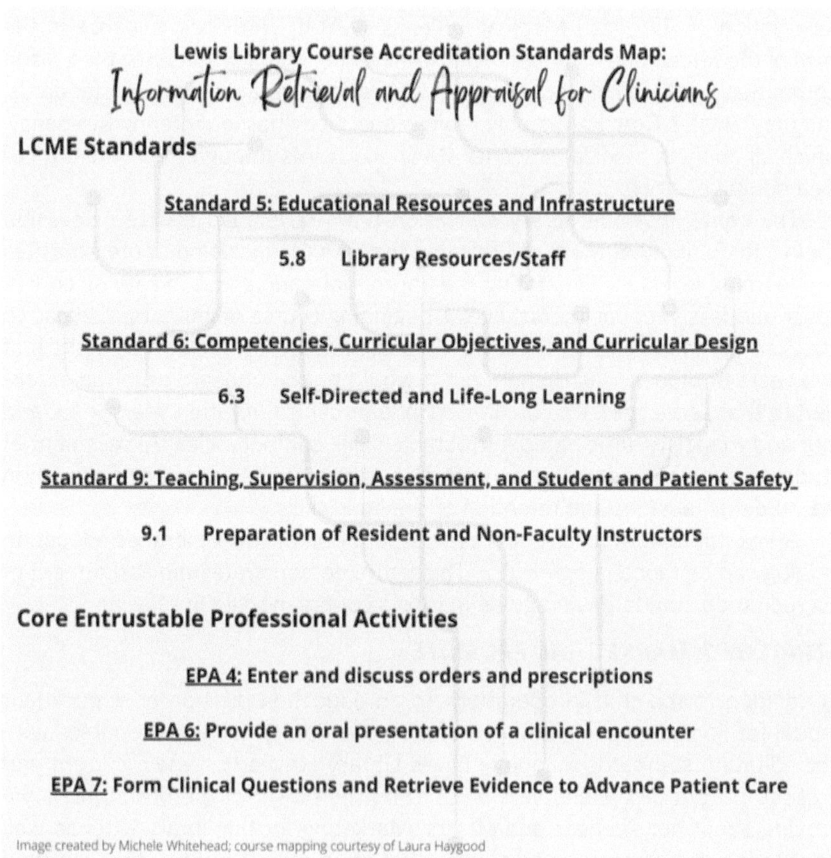

Figure 11.2. Image by Michele Whitehead

that includes not only the context in which learners may want to utilize specific tools but also the advanced skills to refine searching and results.

It is important to note that this type of transition in libraries does not happen overnight, as it becomes the process for recruitment and hiring and organizational or departmental cultural acceptance and buy-in, and it can also include teaching that takes place in a community engagement or health information outreach setting. Librarians with primary duties in consumer health/community engagement and clinical engagement librarians also participate in evolution under this model, and the majority have graduate degrees in education or teaching experience at the university level in an academic discipline.

Building a catalog of course offerings with accreditation standards and guidelines mapping also takes time and investment, but standards and competencies are often easy to identify and include. One example would be the variety of standards and guidelines to consider for medical students. Currently, the Association of American Medical Colleges (AAMC) provides guidance in the form of the fifteen Core Competencies for Entering Medical Students, the Liaison Committee on Medical Education's (LCME's) twelve accreditation standards, and the AAMC's Core Entrustable Professional Activities for Entering Residency, which all apply to medical students at various points through the continuum of their education at HSC.

The content of one library education team-developed course or session could satisfy many of these at the same time, so the inclusion of prerequisites and learning levels for illustrating the appropriate audiences in catalog course descriptions is of equal importance. A beginning course might naturally map to the Core Competencies for Entering Medical Students and be offered in the first two years of didactic instruction, but it would not be unheard of for an extension to that same course to be offered in later clinical rotation years three and four and to satisfy anticipated entrustable skills competencies. Assessment of student learning in advanced courses also requires measurement of growth in the students' abilities and retention of previous skills.

An example from a current course description in Lewis Library's education catalog can be found in figure 11.2. This figure demonstrates the assignment of accreditation standards and guidelines to a course module or offering.

STRATEGY 3: MARKET AND PROMOTE

In addition to the shift in operations to an education division or department model for library teaching and completion of a library catalog of courses with accreditation standards mapping, Lewis Library strives to remain current and present in front of stakeholders by utilizing the power of the descriptions we provide about our services and efforts. Marketing for the library extends well beyond the use of social media, even though in many settings, this can be a beneficial tool. As numerous years' worth of student satisfaction data has shown, very few students on the HSC campus regularly use social media as a primary means of communication. The efforts in shifting toward a better way of connecting and describing how Lewis Library supports accreditation provides very little actual utility if they exist internally or in a library silo, so the importance of marketing and promotion of the library's role in accreditation cannot be overestimated.

Simple suggestions can make an impact related to marketing and the promotion of accreditation-related information. One approach currently popular in website and library subject or research guide design is to highlight accomplishments in a "By the Numbers" data visualization section on the main page.[6] This can be a graphically interesting summary feature where emphasis on data related to the use of library space and feedback leading to renovations or improvements has been incorporated to highlight how the library works to better serve the student body and accommodate more students. This access to appropriate student study space is included as a requirement by health sciences accrediting bodies, and it is an even better scenario when libraries can easily articulate interpretation of data about the availability and how many people utilize these spaces. Three data points Lewis Library includes on the website include an annual gate count, number of full classes taught, and student study space square footage.

Another specific marketing strategy is to provide succinct, but impactful, information in front of department leaders and deans at the least on an annual basis. In the larger administrative process, this may take the form of an informative budget proposal presentation, but opportunities to market do not have to only take place in these formal settings. Creating something as simple as an infographic that highlights new courses designed with accreditation standards and guidelines mapping, space and access updates, and similar data is helpful in not only furthering the library's value message but also for

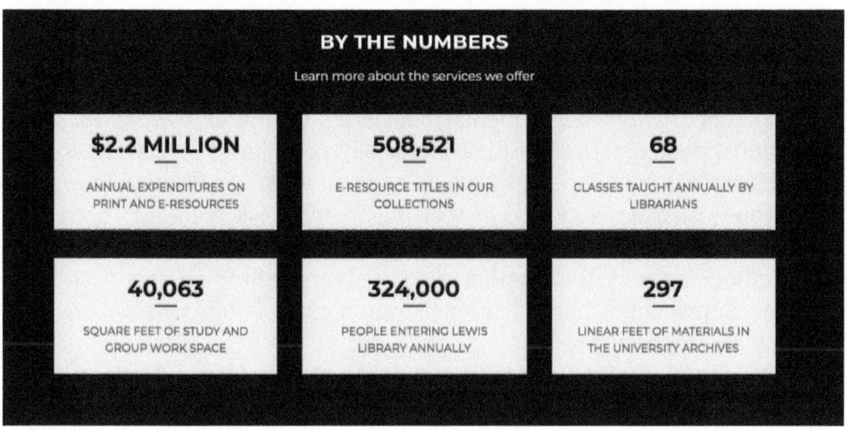

Figure 11.3. Image courtesy of Gibson D. Lewis Health Science Library

reminding busy health sciences leaders that when accreditation reviewer response time comes, the library likely already has the information needed to answer questions.

If librarians and library team members are charged with or take initiative to draft some of these updates, it can also assist in refreshing the memories of library administration of all the areas of work responsibility and task management team members must undertake so library leaders may advocate for librarian inclusion and contributions in the preparation for accreditation reviews. When there is an opportunity for the library to be included in external public-facing marketing and news communications, developing a relationship with campus marketing departments or divisions can also help reinforce the library's value in the academic/scholarship mission and as a necessary space for learning activities to take place. In the hospital setting, HSC library employees have been able to deploy educational advertising and short snippets of the best research tips and tricks because the marketing and communications division is one of the only units with the ability to disseminate communications hospital-wide and direct to practitioners (see figure 11.3).

STRATEGY 4: GO OUTSIDE: PROFESSIONAL DEVELOPMENT OUTSIDE OF LIBRARIES

Librarian attendance at what might be considered nontraditional library meetings, including regional or national meetings related to assessment and accreditation, are important components in the modern professional development of health sciences librarians. One advantage on the HSC campus that may not be generalizable in other settings is that the smaller size of the student body and access to full-time faculty allow librarians to develop involved working relationships within the departments.

Beyond inclusion in committees to hire new faculty or executives on both the academic health sciences campus and hospital, interactions with student organizations and activities, and invitations to departmental retreats and awards banquets, librarians often receive invitations and sponsorships or financial support from departments themselves to attend discipline-specific professional conferences. The library typically contributes to travel support, but departments are consistently encouraging of librarians wanting to expand their professional development in their fields and have mentored both new and seasoned librarians by working as collaborators for projects to submit for presentation. In the hospital setting, Lewis Library team members have been accepted to present at hospital administration conferences, where many discussions of standards emerge.

Often changes in accreditation standards are the focus of research and inquiry first presented in professional meeting settings. In attending conferences such as the American Association of Colleges of Pharmacy (AACP), for example, librarians benefit in a variety of ways. Professional organizations like

AACP have dedicated groups of librarians that are often but not always part of the Medical Library Association (MLA) Drug Information groups. The overlap between the two professional society "worlds" provides librarians attending a pharmacy conference with connections to others with the same responsibilities and performing the same tasks in similar settings. This powerful networking opportunity provides librarians with the information they need for resource consideration and purchasing, discipline-specific strategies in education, and examples of the development of new services for specific audiences.

Another advantage in attending discipline-specific conferences is the opportunity to network and interact with professionals in these fields who often will serve as accreditation reviewers or members of review teams. Building a rapport with professionals in health sciences disciplines eases the stress of accreditation renewal because librarians not only have a sense of what questions to anticipate but also are immediately recognized as being invested in the success of their institutions' programs, because they tried to immerse in the needs of those programs. In hospitals where library roles can take on something less traditional, in-patient care rounding or serving as clinical informationists, clinical professionals have a greater opportunity to see the competence and expertise of these professionals outside of the rapid-paced, fluid patient care environment.

With the transition to virtual meetings in recent years in response to the COVID-19 pandemic and subsequent institutional travel restrictions, many librarians can consider taking advantage of the often-reduced rates for registration in professional conferences and attend these meetings while remaining at home. In libraries where travel support is limited or not provided or in the case of many hospitals with a library team of one, hybrid conference models with virtual components may present a way for librarians to attend and grow their understanding of accreditation without extensive time away or personal expense.

STRATEGY 5: LEARN MORE: ADVANCED DEVELOPMENT

Like the advantages that librarians and library administrators enjoy by attending discipline-specific conferences for the schools or colleges they work closely with, there is also an opportunity for continued involvement in accreditation by attending conferences that enhance understanding of the accreditation process for institutions and assessment. This can be critical for library leaders in the health sciences because of the avenue it provides in working closely with assessment and accreditation teams. The following bulleted list is not exhaustive but provides some examples of advanced professional education opportunities library leaders and senior staff might consider as beneficial to their long-term involvement in institutional and department accreditation:

- Council for Higher Education Accreditation (CHEA)
- Council for Advancement of Standards in Higher Education (CAS)

- American Educational Research Association (AERA)
- American Evaluation Association
- SXSW EDU
- EDUCAUSE

STRATEGY 6: BE ACCOUNTABLE: PROFESSIONAL RESPONSIBILITY

Librarians staying current with their institutions' programs, including in their sustained accreditation efforts, extend beyond education and should be seen as part of a health sciences librarian's professional responsibilities. One way to establish and reinforce this is to set expectations and requirements for liaisons in working with their programs on accreditation.

A common standard found in most public services health sciences library job descriptions is the responsibility to serve as a departmental liaison to specific programs or a subject expert. Often these roles are delegated among librarians with other broader responsibilities. In health sciences libraries with smaller total full-time employees (FTEs), it is not uncommon for librarians in technical services to also be assigned to work closely, building a relationship with faculty and understanding the components of their curriculum and requirements of their programs.

It is important in onboarding and training new librarians that expectations about the responsibilities they have in working with departments be clear. The support of these academic units in the accreditation process should be communicated as part of the librarian's professional responsibilities. Often there should be general standards set forth by library leadership, including the expectation that librarians stay in regular contact with their departments and provide updates to departmental leadership as appropriate.

To build and sustain successful relationships with departments, librarians may use several strategies. Lewis Library has found great success in requesting permission to sit in as nonvoting members or guest attendees of curriculum committees, education councils, and the faculty senate.

The education council in the school of biomedical sciences (SBS) meets monthly to determine faculty appointments, approve proposals for the development of new courses, and review the curriculum as it aligns with accreditation standards. The library has been listed on a standing agenda entry with this group for over a decade to share library-related updates, but the true value in participating in these meetings lies in understanding the requirements for making sure the programs maintain their accreditation and in offering the opportunity for librarians to share the courses, services, and spaces we are developing or revising to support these efforts. With predictable regularity, having this literal seat at the table also keeps the librarian working with the department aware of their responsibilities for communication and accountable for knowing their program intimately well.

STRATEGY 7: MAINTAIN RECORDS THAT COUNT: INSTITUTIONAL AND DEPARTMENTAL HISTORY

Libraries and library staff in the health sciences often have an opportunity to be part of the records management process, from compliance training related to the unique considerations when dealing specifically with health-related records, patient privacy, and research data, to the responsibilities in record keeping to meet federal, state, or private school requirements. Some library professionals in academic and hospital settings also serve as records managers, copyright officers, or in other similar capacities that create and implement systems for maintaining records, developing workflows following requirements of state and federal governments, ensuring the campus stakeholders are following institutional rules and regulations, and signing off on the proper disposition of records as needed. Much of this records management can reveal important information that is useful in the continued or renewal accreditation processes.

The library has a role in the creation of and access to records that can be helpful in accreditation renewals, and one example in Lewis Library was born from the crafting of a library description for grant writers. This document lives publicly on the library's website and was drafted to address very specific information often requested as part of a grant application, but there are similarities in these data points in questions asked by accrediting bodies too.

Institutional leadership can easily point accreditation reviewers to this information, for the library to answer many of the general questions they may have upfront, saving the more granular questions for the reviewers' time interacting with library leaders. Some of the information intentionally included in this description for Lewis Library are elements such as the amount of physical space dedicated for student use and the days and hours the space is accessible, how electronic resources are provided to students and what systems are used, how users of resources can authenticate and gain access to these resources, and the educational opportunities available to support using these tools. Additionally, a library description can include the number of FTE library staff, the hours-of-service provision, and details about everything from borrowing to remote or virtual service options.

This type of document is a starting place where libraries can anticipate the questions reviewers would have based on accreditation guidelines, requirements, and standards. Libraries should set a schedule to review and update these descriptions as changes take place. The recommendation for review is at least twice annually, and Lewis Library's local practice is scheduled by library administration for review in the fall and spring semesters.

Another strength in maintaining records with thought to accreditation purposes that libraries do not always highlight are scholarly repositories and archives or special collections. In addition to the curation of key news items by keeping regular meetings with campus-level marketing and communications groups and diligent efforts to refine collection policies, library archives and repositories are often resources for the institutional memory and to highlight the expertise, quality, and productivity of faculty. Faculty profile systems and repositories can support the dissemination of biographical information about faculty and staff researchers, which supplements information accreditation review teams will request.

STRATEGY 8: STAY FLEXIBLE AND PLAN FOR THE FUTURE WITH BUSINESS CONTINUITY AND SUCCESSION PLANNING

To ensure libraries stay involved in the accreditation conversations of their institutions and programs, there are lessons learned particularly during the COVID-19 pandemic that also apply more broadly to keeping schools on track and the role libraries fulfill. As current library leaders learn more strategies to remain flexible during times of uncertainty, the benefit of devoting energy to staying involved with updates and changes related to accreditation standards is that it provides order or a break from attention disproportionately given to external chaos. Accreditation standards are predictable and prescriptive, and devoting energy to processes and successes in meeting required milestones serves to balance attention from other situations involving more unpredictable changes.

Another important consideration that leaders and educators should devote some energy toward understanding is that in situations where the delivery method of curriculum changes substantially, such as has been the case in shifting to completely virtual or remote learning for clinical didactic and skills instruction, review of accreditation standards becomes even more important in planning and execution of teaching and learning with modalities that have been less familiar. For libraries, this educational shift is important, but there are also implications for collection management and accessibility. Libraries that still operate largely in print monograph and journal holdings may have already learned about the scramble to acquire sufficient electronic resources to support student and faculty needs. For libraries that previously have not operated with a more flexible mindset, this becomes part of a necessary cultural shift.

The training process for professional library staff is one area that merits some discussion as well. Generally, new librarians should be trained to understand the accreditation processes for the schools or colleges they work with and the overall institutional requirements and requirements of other programs. Novice librarians benefit from understanding the roles of accreditation bodies, the responsibilities of the institution, and the library's responsibilities even when the standards do not explicitly utilize language that includes the word "library."

Continuity and succession planning have also been revealed to be extremely important, because the institutional memory does help ensure avoidance of previous pitfalls, and librarians with experience in accreditation review should document those experiences and the questions asked by reviewers and prepare newer library team members for what those experiences may entail. Library leaders and mid-level managers can include librarians in the review experience with primary responsibility to first observe or contribute to one targeted area, such as sharing more about the curriculum development process, to familiarize more team members in what to anticipate should they be tasked to fulfill this role in the future.

CONCLUSION

In this chapter, the author described eight strategies that have proven successful in staying involved in accreditation processes in both academic and hospital health sciences settings. Librarians and library team members who can clearly demonstrate how their work contributes to sustained success not only represent their libraries well but ensure involvement in other spaces where their expertise may be underutilized. In the future, considering libraries as a value-add, the knowledge and experience information professionals can bring because of their work in accreditation may lead to the ability to grow program offerings and rise above competitors in the health sciences. The author encourages library team members and leaders to make the extra effort to embrace a sometimes nontraditional, multidisciplinary approach in staying the course for accreditation.

NOTES

1. R. Cullen, M. Clark, and R. Esson, "Evidence-Based Information-Seeking Skills of Junior Doctors Entering the Workforce: An Evaluation of the Impact of Information Literacy Training During Pre-Clinical Years," *Health Information and Libraries Journal* 28, no. 2 (2011): 119–29, https://doi.org/10.1111/j.1471-1842.2011.00933.x
2. "The Joint Commission Accreditation Milestones," accessed December 2021, https://www.jointcommission.org/accreditation-and-certification/accredited/accreditation-milestones/.
3. Juliana Kaplan, "The Psychologist Who Coined the Phrase the 'Great Resignation' Reveals How He Saw It Coming and Where He Sees It Going," accessed November 28, 2021, https://www.businessinsider.com/why-everyone-is-quitting-great-resignation-psychologist-pandemic-rethink-life-2021-10.
4. Southern Association of Colleges and Schools Commission on Colleges, "About SACSCOC," accessed January 3, 2022, https://sacscoc.org.
5. Association of College and Research Libraries, *Framework for Information Literacy for Higher Education*, accessed November 26, 2021, https://www.ala.org/acrl/sites/ala.org.acrl/files/content/issues/infolit/framework1.pdf.
6. "Data Visualization in Web Design: 12 Stunning Examples," accessed January 3, 2022, https://designshack.net/articles/graphics/data-visualization-web-design-examples/.

BIBLIOGRAPHY

Association of College and Research Libraries. *Framework for Information Literacy for Higher Education.* Accessed November 26, 2021. https://www.ala.org/acrl/sites/ala.org.acrl/files/content/issues/infolit/framework1.pdf.

Cullen, R., M. Clark, and R. Esson. "Evidence-Based Information-Seeking Skills of Junior Doctors Entering the Workforce: An Evaluation of the Impact of Information Literacy Training during Pre-Clinical Years." *Health Information and Libraries Journal* 28, no. 2 (2011): 119–29. https://doi.org/10.1111/j.1471-1842.2011.00933.x.

"Data Visualization in Web Design: 12 Stunning Examples." Accessed January 3, 2022. https://designshack.net/articles/graphics/data-visualization-web-design-examples/.

Kaplan, Juliana. "The Psychologist Who Coined the Phrase the 'Great Resignation' Reveals How He Saw It Coming and Where He Sees It Going." Accessed November 28, 2021. https://www.businessinsider.com/why-everyone-is-quitting-great-resignation-psychologist-pandemic-rethink-life-2021-10.

Southern Association of Colleges and Schools Commission on Colleges. "About SACSCOC." Accessed January 3, 2022. https://sacscoc.org.

"The Joint Commission Accreditation Milestones." Accessed December 2021. https://www.jointcommission.org/accreditation-and-certification/accredited/accreditation-milestones/.

12

Librarian Involvement in a School of Medicine Accreditation Initiative

ASSESSING INFORMATION-SEEKING SKILLS DURING CURRICULAR SELF-DIRECTED LEARNING ACTIVITIES

Douglas L. Varner, Grant Connors, Yvonne M. Hernandez, Jeff Weinfeld, G. Ian Gallicano, Jett McCann, Georgetown University

The Georgetown University School of Medicine (SOM) successfully completed a Liaison Committee on Medical Education (LCME) accreditation evaluation in February 2019. As part of the postsurvey monitoring update, the LCME required that the SOM address Accreditation Standard 6, Element 6.3, mandating the assessment of information-seeking skills relating to self-directed learning. This requirement has been embedded into an ongoing SOM continuous quality improvement (CQI) process to incorporate Element 6.3 into the preclinical curriculum. This chapter will discuss self-directed learning activities identified in the SOM curriculum based on the LCME requirement and the CQI process, how faculty collaborated with librarians on the application of a preestablished assessment tool to measure information-seeking behaviors during self-directed learning activities and provided feedback to the students on sources consulted and search strategies used for the self-directed learning activity.

An overview of self-directed learning, including definitions, applications, and assessment of this learning modality, will also be discussed.

OVERVIEW OF SELF-DIRECTED LEARNING

WHAT IS SELF-DIRECTED LEARNING?

Malcolm Knowles is generally considered to be the pioneer in proposing self-directed learning as an instructional modality and defined the term as "a process in which individuals take the initiative, with or without the help of others, in diagnosing their learning needs, formulating learning goals, identifying human and material resources for learning, choosing and implementing appropriate learning strategies, and evaluating learning outcomes."[1]

The International Society for Self-Directed Learning further defines self-directed learning as "an intentional learning process that is created and evaluated by the learner."[2]

Garrison outlines a theoretical model for self-directed learning composed of the following elements: self-management, focusing on the social and behavioral implementation of learning intentions, followed by self-monitoring, which addresses cognitive and metacognitive processes. The final element of the model involves learner motivation revolving around the initiation and maintenance of efforts toward learning and the achievement of cognitive goals.[3]

In a further assessment and evaluation of the theoretical model, Brandt proposes "autonomy" as an additional element of the model.[4] Autonomy is defined as the ability to recognize available choices, take charge of one's learning, and control choices through ongoing reflection and evaluation.[5]

Brandt further describes self-directed learning as a process that evolves organically as a generalized methodology in the progression of the student's academic growth in addition to being discipline specific, transferring across multiple fields of study.[6]

SELF-DIRECTED LEARNING IN MEDICAL EDUCATION

Malcolm Knowles, the previously mentioned pioneer in the field of self-directed learning, outlines the importance of self-directed learning in the health sciences in the description of a pilot program at the University of Southern California, in which the primary focus of the study is the development and implementation of self-directed learning activities for physician learning.[7] The pilot program at the University of Southern California consisted of three program components: the development of a brief, but formal, learning plan customized to the individual; information brokering in which a medical librarian linked participating physicians to appropriate teaching/learning resources; and peer resources groups in which participants could engage in information sharing, problem solving, technical assistance, and informal personal interaction.[8] Knowles goes on to describe the volatile nature or "half-life" of knowledge, skills, attitudes, and values required by physicians, nurses, allied health professionals, and pharmacists.[9]

Self-directed learning is described as an essential component of medical education due to the expansion of knowledge, accessibility to information, and enhanced emphasis on reflection.[10]

Heck and colleagues describe how the rapid turnover of medical information results in ever-expanding content within the undergraduate medical curriculum while the window of time to cover this content in the curricular calendar remains constant.[11] This phenomenon leads to the increasing importance for medical students to have skills in self-directed learning.[12]

SELF-DIRECTED LEARNING IN NURSING EDUCATION

Self-directed learning has come to the forefront in nursing education as a teaching methodology and pedagogy.

Cadorin and colleagues describe self-directed learning skills development as an essential prerequisite for both nursing students and nurses to proactively address the ongoing challenges in the practice of healthcare.[13]

Chakkaravarthy and colleagues propose that the increased complexities in healthcare settings demand that nurses and midwives become involved in lifelong learning by means of self-directed learning to ensure the delivery of quality healthcare.[14]

SELF-DIRECTED LEARNING IN DENTAL EDUCATION

A review spearheaded by the American Dental Education Association, Commission on Change and Innovation in Dental Education discusses the importance of benchmarking in the development of problem solving, critical thinking, and self-directed learning as dental school graduates evolve into expert performers in the years after matriculating from degree-granting programs in dental education.[15]

ASSESSMENT OF SELF-DIRECTED LEARNING AND BARRIERS TO IMPLEMENTATION

A randomized, controlled trial videorecorded surgical residents performing an intestinal anastomosis on cadaveric pig bowel. A second videorecording of the residents performing the procedure was evaluated by two attending surgeons, comparing the intervention group who had viewed a video of an expert performing the anastomosis to the control group who did not view the expert video.[16] The results showed that the intervention group did not perform statistically significantly better than residents in the control group.[17] However, the researchers discussed the small sample size as a limitation of the study, noted positive feedback for the expert video from members of the intervention group, and felt that there is a role for e-learning and video as an instructional modality vehicle to deliver self-directed learning content in the future training of surgical residents.[18]

A scoping review conducted in Canada examining physicians' use of self-directed learning for continuing medical education found that the facilitators and barriers to the use of self-directed learning in support of continuing education activities included physicians' time constraints, access to tools, teamwork and collaborative work, and perception of the content of the self-directed learning program—all factors that can influence physician engagement in self-directed learning.[19]

Murad and colleagues conducted a systematic review and found that evidence suggests self-directed learning in health professions education is associated with moderate improvement in the knowledge domain compared with traditional teaching methods and may be as effective in the skills domain.[20] Skills domains are defined as the physical demonstration of learned content, and attitudes domains are comprised of the learner receiving, responding, valuing, organizing, and internalizing learned content.[21]

Hill and colleagues conducted a survey evaluating the feasibility and effectiveness of a self-directed learning activity in a six-week infectious disease module for a first-year medical student course. Results indicate that students strongly agreed that the exercise contributed to learning new clinical knowledge (92 percent), and contributed to the acquisition of lifelong learning skills (85 percent).[22] Hill recommends that self-directed learning assignments occur regularly throughout the preclinical curriculum to promote lifelong learning skills, that self-directed learning assignments can be successfully implemented in preclinical courses and are valued by the students as contributing to the skills necessary for delivery of effective patient care.[23]

Ricotta and colleagues postulate that while the majority of assessments of self-directed learning in medical education should be formative, summative assessments are important during rotations for students in learning environments with enhanced autonomy and at transition points in the curriculum in which students need to demonstrate competency to move to the next level of independence.[24] Ricotta and colleagues further state that appropriate assessment modalities and strategies need to be established and refined to foster self-directed learning as a fundamental competency for healthcare professionals.[25]

A survey that measured faculty needs assessment for fostering self-directed learning found that while there was overwhelming agreement that physicians in training should be self-directed learners, faculty require training in education approaches to promote self-directed learning.[26]

LIAISON COMMITTEE ON MEDICAL EDUCATION AND SELF-DIRECTED LEARNING

DESCRIPTION OF LIAISON COMMITTEE ON MEDICAL EDUCATION MANDATE

Medical education programs leading to the MD degree in the United States and Canada are accredited by the Liaison Committee on Medical Education (LCME). LCME accreditation is a voluntary, peer-reviewed process of quality assurance that determines whether the medical education program meets established standards. This process also fosters institutional and programmatic improvement.[27]

To achieve and maintain accreditation, a medical education program leading to the MD degree in the United States and Canada must meet the LCME accreditation standards contained in the LCME document *Functions and Structure of a Medical School*.[28]

In 2004, the Liaison Committee on Medical Education endorsed medical college accreditation standards that promote medical students' skills acquisition in self-directed learning, increasing the interest in and emphasis on exploring this process in the medical education literature.[29]

The LCME Accreditation Element 6.3 specifically addresses curricular integration of self-directed learning activities: The faculty of a medical school ensure that the medical curriculum includes self-directed learning experiences and unscheduled time to allow medical students to develop the skills of lifelong learning. Self-directed learning involves medical students' self-assessment of learning needs; independent identification, analysis, and synthesis of relevant information; appraisal of the credibility of information sources; and feedback on these skills.[30]

The LCME defines self-directed learning as including all of the following components as a single unified sequence that occurs over a relatively short time: (1) the medical student's self-assessment of his/her learning needs; (2) the medical student's independent identification, analysis, and synthesis of relevant information; (3) the medical student's appraisal of the credibility of information sources; and (4) the facilitator's assessment of and feedback to the student on his/her information-seeking skills.[31]

LCME standards promote the delivery of an integrated and coordinated curriculum that is designed to develop the skills of self-directed independent study in medical students.

This LCME standard requires the inclusion of unscheduled time and independent learning components "to allow medical students to develop the skills of lifelong learning."[32] As medical students transition to lifelong learners, medical educators continue to consider when self-directed learning should become the predominant instructional method.[33]

GEORGETOWN UNIVERSITY SCHOOL OF MEDICINE CURRICULAR OVERVIEW

The Georgetown medical school experience is centered in *cura personalis*—care for a person's psychological, spiritual, and social well-being in addition to their physical well-being. The School of Medicine (SOM) instructional trajectory, known as the Journeys Curriculum, is broken down into three distinct phases: the Foundational Phase, Core Clinical Phase, and Advanced Clinical Phase.

Critical thinking, cognitive integration, and lifelong learning are qualities that are vital to successful medical practice and guide the development of the preclinical phase. The foundational curriculum is divided into six blocks of core content, each followed by a two-week study and exam period. The blocks are organized in a logical progression of organ-system-based modules that integrate basic science disciplines and doctoring training.[34]

EXAMPLES OF SELF-DIRECTED LEARNING IN THE SOM CURRICULUM

Self-directed learning activities are infused throughout the Georgetown University School of Medicine (SOM) curriculum to promote self-reflection of learning inflection points and development of skills to address learning needs. In addition, curricular activities that foster conducting focused searches for resources embedded in the curriculum and extracurricular resources to address learning needs and assess the validity and relevance of resources retrieved to address learning needs provide curricular touchpoints for the students to develop skills that promote lifelong learning as the students progress through their training and professional practice of medicine. The curricular activities outlined in this chapter discuss how the SOM has addressed the LCME-defined goals of leveraging self-directed learning activities in the delivery of course content using an integrated and longitudinal methodology to provide learners with opportunities to independently acquire, analyze, synthesize, and apply knowledge in clinical and research settings.

Librarians at the Dahlgren Memorial Library (DML) participate in three courses in the SOM curriculum in which self-directed learning activities are embedded into the course.

EVIDENCE-BASED MEDICINE LONGITUDINAL PROJECT (YEARS 1 AND 2)

In the evidence-based medicine (EBM) course, students learn to evaluate medical literature and apply evidence from the literature to patient care. Each student completes a longitudinal project that includes all components of self-directed learning and teaches principles of lifelong learning. This project is completed in three staged assignments followed by a student presentation to fellow students and a faculty leader. Throughout the course, the students engage in self-directed learning activities that are facilitated and supported by librarians.

SELF-ASSESSMENT OF STUDENT LEARNING NEEDS

In the first EBM assignment, students identify a disease and treatment that they would like to learn more about, and create a patient scenario that poses a clinical question. This scenario carries through to all the subsequent assignments and the final presentation for the EBM longitudinal course.

INDEPENDENT IDENTIFICATION, ANALYSIS, AND SYNTHESIS OF RELEVANT INFORMATION

In the first assignment, students identify a background question and then search for a narrative review article that would answer their question. They conclude the assignment by asking a patient-focused foreground question that again relates to their clinical scenario.

Before the second assignment, librarians teach a workshop composed of fifteen to seventeen students focusing on clinical literature searches, constructing well-defined and reproducible search strategies, and finding the best type of evidence to answer clinical questions.

The second assignment requires students to format their foreground question into the PICO format (Problem/Patient/Population, Intervention/Indicator, Comparison, Outcome) and then create and execute a literature search in the MEDLINE database using the OVID® interface. Students must find randomized controlled trials (RCTs) that answer their foreground question.

In the third assignment, students choose one of the RCTs they retrieved from the previous assignment that the students evaluate independently and critically. The students submit their evaluation for review by faculty. In preparation for the presentation, the student is asked to find a meta-analysis or Cochrane Systematic Review on the same question, and to read and weigh the additional evidence in comparison to the RCT.

INDEPENDENT AND FACILITATOR APPRAISAL OF THE CREDIBILITY OF INFORMATION SOURCES

For each step, the assignment asks students to evaluate papers from various sources and choose a valid article for their question type. Faculty graders, which include librarians, provide feedback on the paper evaluation, including type of study and its credibility, to students after submission of each of the three assignments. This allows students to modify questions and topics and choose different articles for subsequent assignments.

During the project presentation at the end of the course, students summarize their question and answers and discuss the types of sources identified. They weigh these sources and article types in creating a final answer to their foreground question.

ASSESSMENT AND FEEDBACK ON STUDENT INFORMATION-SEEKING SKILLS

Faculty grade students and provide narrative feedback at multiple steps throughout the project, including on the background question and article, on the search for randomized control trials, and on the evaluation of the RCT. After submitting the literature search, each student receives detailed feedback on their search strategy, which assesses the student's information-seeking skills. At the end of the final assignment, students present their findings to peers and faculty in a small group setting. Students receive verbal feedback from other students and faculty regarding information sources and their overall process for finding an answer. The presentation is graded using a rubric with narrative feedback from faculty submitted via Canvas. This assignment directly satisfies LCME Accreditation Element 6.3, mandating the assessment of information-seeking skills relating to self-directed learning.

MEDICAL STUDENT GRAND ROUNDS (YEARS 1 AND 2)

Medical student grand rounds (MSGR) is a longitudinal course that meets once or twice per year during the first three years in the SOM curriculum. The learning objectives related to self-directed learning are as follows:

- Work cooperatively in groups to discuss and solve a clinical problem.
- Identify which information is relevant to a clinical problem.
- Interpret clinical clues based on history and physical exam.
- Incorporate scientific data from the medical literature into clinical problem solving and assess the validity, accuracy, and authenticity of the studies consulted.

Students work in groups of four to answer questions related to a clinical problem. They receive information about a medical case progressively over a one-week period of time and are tasked to formulate a differential diagnosis, interpret diagnostic tests, and retrieve relevant information to determine what evidence from the literature supports each aspect of the differential diagnosis the student groups construct relevant to the case.

Each group submits answers to the progressive case questions. In most cases, students have not been taught all the material relevant to the clinical problem, so they must identify the symptoms, terminology, diagnostic tests, and results that are unfamiliar, search information on these topics, and identify the resources that are useful to answer the case questions. Students are expected to attend the grand rounds final presentation session fully prepared to discuss relevant aspects of the clinical case with their peers and the faculty panel. On the day of the MSGR, a panel of experts (clinicians, basic scientists, and other healthcare personnel) evaluates and provides a critical assessment of the case in collaboration with students. A moderator facilitates the session.

As part of the MSGR orientation, students receive a presentation from a DML librarian on evidence-based resources that provide evidence summaries, diagnostic support, and drug information. In addition, the librarian provides a demonstration of effective ways to search these resources to answer the MSGR case questions. As part of the case answers they submit, students must indicate the information sources they consulted and the search terms they used to retrieve information from these sources. This information is sent to the library personnel for analysis and feedback. Students are encouraged to seek help from the librarians as they are researching the clinical case.

During the MSGR final presentation, students are called on in their groups to answer case questions within the large group session, where they receive feedback from the panelists and moderator. In addition, library staff provide an analysis of the students' information-seeking skills, a critical assessment of the resources used and feedback on how to improve their search strategy development skills. In this critical assessment of resources consulted for the MSGR case, the librarians provide teaching points that instruct the students on how to differentiate the value and robustness of information found from generalized sources on the internet, consumer health resources, and peer-reviewed, authoritative, scholarly professional resources. Although this method does not provide individual feedback to students, it does reinforce to all the best practices for finding high-quality clinical sources. Library staff track the progress of the class over time to identify improvements and gaps as the students continually improve their literature search skills and critical appraisal abilities. This assignment directly addresses LCME Accreditation Element 6.3, mandating the assessment of information-seeking skills relating to self-directed learning.

MEDICAL EMBRYOLOGY MINI-LITERATURE REVIEW PAPER (YEAR 1)

The medical embryology course is a longitudinal course that begins in year 1 of the SOM curriculum and continues through year 2. During the portion of the medical embryology courses that occurs in the reproduction module during the spring of the first year of the SOM curriculum, students are assigned to work in groups and to conduct a literature review on a selected topic related to sexual development and reproduction, access the information retrieved from the literature review, and synthesize that information into a paper. The goals of the assignment are formulated so that the students collaborate with peers to author a publication-quality manuscript on a chosen clinical or basic science research topic relating to embryology and to critique a peer group's manuscript using a detailed rubric. The latter part of the assignment mimics the peer-review process conducted prior to a paper being published in a scientific journal.

Prior to the start of the assignment, students view a literature search tutorial followed by completion of an assessment in the form of an interactive, summative quiz administered through Canvas. Both the literature search tutorial and the quiz are developed by DML librarians. The students then apply what they learn in the tutorial in a literature search workshop taught by DML librarians. During the workshop, students engage in hands-on activities designed to teach how to effectively search scientific and medical literature using best practices for conducting searches in Ovid® MEDLINE and learn to assess the quality of these sources using criteria such as the journal impact factor, currency of the content, and rigor of the peer-review process for the sources. As students start researching their topics, each student must complete a self-directed learning worksheet and submit the worksheet for review by the DML librarians, who provide individual feedback to students on their search strategies and their appraisal of information sources. The worksheet assessment tool is shown in the appendix and was adapted from a model used at the University of Illinois College of Medicine. DML librarians, SOM faculty, and administrators collaborated in the adaption of the assessment tool and the customization of the tool to fit the unique needs of the SOM curriculum. Students also complete a tutorial with an assessment in the form of an interactive, summative quiz on academic writing that covers academic integrity and misconduct, plagiarism, and managing citations.

SELF-ASSESSMENT OF STUDENT LEARNING NEEDS

Depending on their interests, each group of three to four students chooses their research topic from an extensive list of acceptable topics or can propose a new topic with approval of the medical embryology course director. Although students write the review paper as a group, each individual student must fill out the self-directed learning worksheet identifying a learning gap that they want to research for the paper.

INDEPENDENT IDENTIFICATION, ANALYSIS, AND SYNTHESIS OF RELEVANT INFORMATION

Throughout the weeks of the assignment, students identify and analyze up to thirty quality references relevant to their review paper. Early in the process, students submit the self-directed learning worksheet detailing the search terms they used to research their knowledge gap, identifying the sources where they found relevant information, listing relevant citations of primary sources, and analyzing one of the sources for its strengths and weaknesses in addressing the knowledge gap. The students submit the self-directed learning worksheet to the librarians for review and formative feedback.

INDEPENDENT AND FACILITATOR APPRAISAL OF THE CREDIBILITY OF INFORMATION SOURCES

The self-directed learning worksheet includes a rubric given to students that the librarians use to assess students' search strategy, information sources, and analysis of the sources. The worksheet also contains a section for librarians to provide narrative feedback to each student.

To complete the worksheet students are asked to

- state the topic of the paper (again a topic related to embryology);
- identify a learning gap;
- list sources used to address the learning gap originating from peer-reviewed and professional resources;
- list search strategies used to retrieve information on the paper topic; and
- identify three relevant citations retrieved from the search strategy.

Students are then asked to select one of the retrieved articles and evaluate the paper's strengths, weaknesses, and whether the article provided information to address the learning gap.

Students are evaluated by librarians on each of these criteria according to a scale that assesses the students as

- needing improvement on the specific point,
- meeting expectations, or
- exceeding expectations.

The full worksheet outlining the above elements is included in the appendix.

Each student receives individual feedback either through an online consultation meeting or asynchronously through Canvas. The synchronous exercise is designed so that the individual feedback provided by the librarians is conveyed in a group setting to all members of the writing group during the session so that the group members may learn and benefit from the individual student assessments. After the library consultation, students decide as a group which sources to include in the paper. Using these references, the student groups collaborate to produce a focused manuscript on a contemporary development in a specific area relating to embryology. Each student contributes to the synthesis of the information, the discussion of the findings, and the writing of the manuscript.

ASSESSMENT AND FEEDBACK ON STUDENT INFORMATION-SEEKING SKILLS

Students receive formative feedback on their information-seeking skills early in the planning and writing process as described above. After submission of the paper, the papers are de-identified and randomly assigned to a peer group for critiquing and evaluation. Students follow a points-based rubric provided by the course director, which requires the students to write narrative feedback and rationales for the scores they assign. The rubric includes assessment of the credibility and quality of the information sources used, the organization of the paper, synthesis of the content, and clarity of the arguments. The information skills that are reinforced during the librarian-facilitated synchronous/asynchronous consultations serve as a guide for students to assess the work of their peers. Groups are directed to provide constructive criticism and feedback throughout the project—both within their group during manuscript writing and to the group whose paper they are evaluating. In addition to evaluating another group's paper, students evaluate each other within the group using a scaled score, and provide narrative feedback on the level and quality of their peer's contribution to the assignment. The student writing groups have the ability to initiate a rebuttal process after review of their peer group evaluation comments if concerns or disagreements arise regarding the peer group comments on the paper. The course director provides quality control by reviewing a number of the papers, particularly when students submit a rebuttal to the reviewers.

STUDENT EVALUATION OF THE SELF-DIRECTED LEARNING ACTIVITY IN THE MEDICAL EMBRYOLOGY COURSE

Students provided overall comments that the synchronous or asynchronous feedback during the librarian-facilitated self-directed learning activity was helpful. There were concerns relating to the fast turnaround for student completion of the worksheet, the necessity for the students to attend the synchronous sessions on short notice, posing difficulty in attendance, and the timing of the feedback that occurred after the students had completed their search strategies and assessment of relevant articles for inclusion in the review. The medical embryology course directors and curricular managers have scheduled the librarian-facilitated synchronous self-directed learning assessment activities during the second week of the medical embryology course, and the feedback from the librarians is timed to coincide with the point in the research trajectory when the students are gathering and assessing relevant articles for inclusion in the paper. Lastly, an assessment will be conducted of the learning points discussed in the librarian-facilitated workshop and the self-directed learning activity to minimize redundancy of content covered in both these learning interventions.

POSITIVE OUTCOMES OF THE SELF-DIRECTED LEARNING ACTIVITY IN THE MEDICAL EMBRYOLOGY COURSE

The self-directed learning activity in the medical embryology course provided the students with librarian intervention and feedback at the "point-of-need"; the students were writing and completing tasks to satisfy a curricular requirement. Perceived positive outcomes of librarian involvement in this effort include the following:

- Direct librarian involvement and contribution to a required accreditation mandate: LCME Accreditation Element 6.3, addressing the assessment of information-seeking skills relating to self-directed learning.

- The provision of a teachable moment in the SOM curriculum in which the librarians are able to demonstrate to the students the importance of information-seeking behavior to enhance curriculum-mandated self-directed learning activities and development of lifelong learning habits.
- Demonstration to students of the use of the appropriate information resources to fill a knowledge gap (i.e., the use of MEDLINE instead of non-validated sources such as Google or Wikipedia).
- Librarian expertise integrated and woven into this entire process to provide a real-time and just-in-time assessment of information-seeking and critical appraisal skills in students applied using a self-directed learning strategy.

This effort enhanced the visibility of the librarians to both faculty and students and generated positive feedback from faculty and administrators.

CONCLUSION

This chapter provided a current snapshot of knowledge on the definitions, applications, curriculum integration, and assessment of self-directed learning activities. An outline of the Liaison Committee on Medical Education (LCME) mandate for the incorporation of self-directed learning activities was provided with a focus on assessing information seeking, critical appraisal, and development of lifelong learning skills. A description of the Georgetown University School of Medicine curricular organization and underlying foundations in the learner-centric course of study and modular organization of learning content was provided, as well as three examples of self-directed learning activities embedded in the SOM medicine curriculum. The vital role librarians play in the LCME-mandated administration and assessment of self-directed learning activities was also highlighted. Particular emphasis is placed on librarian involvement in the development, administration, and assessment of a self-directed learning worksheet completed by the students in the medical embryology course as the student writing groups are completing their review paper requirement for the course. These librarians developed and implemented touchpoints in the SOM curriculum, provided an important contribution to the overall accreditation process, and directly addressed an important LCME mandate to develop and nurture medical student lifelong learning skills. The LCME has indicated from the provision of feedback and continuing assessment that the SOM has satisfied Accreditation Standard 6, Element 6.3, based on the initiatives undertaken and still developing that have been described in this chapter.

NOTES

1. Malcolm S. Knowles, *Self-Directed Learning: A Guide for Learners and Teachers* (New York: Association Press, 1975), 18.
2. International Society for Self-Directed Learning, "About Us," accessed January 28, 2022, https://www.sdlglobal.com/about-us.

3. D. Randy Garrison, "Self-Directed Learning: Toward a Comprehensive Model," *Adult Education Quarterly* 48, no. 1 (1997): 18–33.
4. W. Christopher Brandt, *Measuring Student Success Skills: A Review of the Literature on Self-Directed Learning. 21st Century Success Skills* (Dover, NH, National Center for the Improvement of Educational Assessment, 2020), http://www.nciea.org.
5. Brandt, *Measuring Student Success Skills*, 5.
6. Brandt, *Measuring Student Success Skills*, 9.
7. Malcolm S. Knowles, "Application in Continuing Education for the Health Professions: Chapter Five of 'Andragogy in Action,'" *Mobius* 5, no. 2 (1985): 80–100, https://doi.org/10.1002/chp.4760050212.
8. Knowles, "Application in Continuing Education," 82.
9. Knowles, "Application in Continuing Education," 80.
10. N. Ainoda, H. Onishi, and Y. Yasuda, "Definitions and Goals of 'Self-Directed Learning' in Contemporary Medical Education Literature," *Annals of the Academy of Medicine, Singapore* 34, no. 8 (2005): 515–19.
11. Amber J. Heck, Courtney E. Cross, and Veronica Y. Tatum, "Early Medical Education Readiness Interventions: Enhancing Undergraduate Preparedness," in *Handbook of Research on the Efficacy of Training Programs and Systems in Medical Education*, ed. Ruth Gotian, Yoon Kang, and Joseph Safdieh (Hershey, PA: IGI Global, 2020), 283–304.
12. Heck, Cross, and Tatum, "Early Medical Education," 287.
13. L. Cadorin, V. Bressan, and A. Palese, "Instruments Evaluating the Self-Directed Learning Abilities among Nursing Students and Nurses: A Systematic Review of Psychometric Properties," *BMC Medical Education* 17, no. 1 (2017): 229-017-1072-73, https://doi.org/10.1186/s12909-017-1072-3.
14. K. Chakkaravarthy et al., "Predictors for Nurses and Midwives' Readiness towards Self-Directed Learning: An Integrated Review," *Nurse Education Today* 69 (October 2018): 60–66, https://doi.org/10.1016/j.nedt.2018.06.030.
15. W. D. Hendricson et al., "Educational Strategies Associated with Development of Problem-Solving, Critical Thinking, and Self-Directed Learning," *Journal of Dental Education* 70, no. 9 (2006): 925–36, https://doi.org/10.1002/j.0022-0337.2006.70.9.tb04163.x.
16. G. Chartrand et al., "Self-Directed Learning by Video as a Means to Improve Technical Skills in Surgery Residents: A Randomized Controlled Trial," *BMC Medical Education* 21, no. 1 (2021): article 91, https://doi.org/10.1186/s12909-021-02524-y.
17. Chartrand et al., "Self-Directed Learning by Video," 7.
18. Chartrand et al., "Self-Directed Learning by Video," 7.
19. D. Jeong et al., "Barriers and Facilitators to Self-Directed Learning in Continuing Professional Development for Physicians in Canada: A Scoping Review," *Academic Medicine: Journal of the Association of American Medical Colleges* 93, no. 8 (2018): 1245–54, https://doi.org/10.1097/ACM.0000000000002237.
20. M. H. Murad et al., "The Effectiveness of Self-Directed Learning in Health Professions Education: A Systematic Review," *Medical Education* 44, no. 11 (2010): 1057–68, https://doi.org/10.1111/j.1365-2923.2010.03750.x.

21. Vector Solutions, "Teaching Attitudes: The Affective Domain of Learning and Learning Objectives," accessed January 28, 2022, https://www.vectorsolutions.com/resources/blogs/teaching-attitudes-the-affective-domain-of-learning-and-learning-objectives/.
22. M. Hill et al., "Implementation and Evaluation of a Self-Directed Learning Activity for First-Year Medical Students," *Medical Education Online* 25, no. 1 (2020): 1717780, https://doi.org/10.1080/10872981.2020.1717780.
23. Hill et al., "Implementation and Evaluation," 6.
24. D. N. Ricotta et al., "Self-Directed Learning in Medical Education: Training for a Lifetime of Discovery," *Teaching and Learning in Medicine* (July 2021): 1–11, https://doi.org/10.1080/10401334.2021.1938074.
25. Ricotta et al., "Self-Directed Learning," 8.
26. Y. S. Lim, V. T. Lyons, and J. M. Willey, "Supporting Self-Directed Learning: A National Needs Analysis," *Medical Science Educator* 31, no. 3 (2021): 1091–99, https://doi.org/10.1007/s40670-021-01278-y.
27. Liaison Committee on Medical Education, "Scope and Purpose of Accreditation," accessed January 28, 2022, https://lcme.org/about/.
28. Liaison Committee on Medical Education, *Functions and Structure of a Medical School: Standards for Accreditation of Medical Education Programs Leading to the MD Degree*. Washington, DC: Association of American Medical Colleges, 2021.
29. F. A. Simon and C. A. Aschenbrener, "Undergraduate Medical Education Accreditation as a Driver of Lifelong Learning," *Journal of Continuing Education in the Health Professions* 25, no. 3 (2005): 157–61, https://doi.org/10.1002/chp.23.
30. Liaison Committee on Medical Education, *Functions and Structure of a Medical School*, 8.
31. Liaison Committee on Medical Education, *Functions and Structure of a Medical School*, 26.
32. J. H. Wu, P. A. Gruppuso, and E. Y. Adashi, "The Self-Directed Medical Student Curriculum," *JAMA* 326, no. 20 (2021): 2005–6, https://doi.org/10.1001/jama.2021.16312.
33. Wu, Gruppuso, and Adashi, "Self-Directed."
34. Georgetown University School of Medicine, "Journeys Curriculum," accessed January 28, 2022, https://som.georgetown.edu/curriculum/journeyscurriculum/.

BIBLIOGRAPHY

Ainoda, N., H. Onishi, and Y. Yasuda. "Definitions and Goals of 'Self-Directed Learning' in Contemporary Medical Education Literature." *Annals of the Academy of Medicine, Singapore* 34, no. 8 (2005): 515–19.

Brandt, W. Christopher. *Measuring Student Success Skills: A Review of the Literature on Self-Directed Learning. 21st Century Success Skills*. Dover, NH: National Center for the Improvement of Educational Assessment, 2020. http://www.nciea.org.

Cadorin, L., V. Bressan, and A. Palese. "Instruments Evaluating the Self-Directed Learning Abilities among Nursing Students and Nurses: A Systematic Review of Psychometric Properties." *BMC Medical Education* 17, no. 1 (2017): 229-017-1072-73. https://doi.org/10.1186/s12909-017-1072-3.

Chakkaravarthy, K., N. Ibrahim, M. Mahmud, and M. R. Venkatasalu. "Predictors for Nurses and Midwives' Readiness towards Self-Directed Learning: An Integrated Review." *Nurse Education Today* 69 (October 2018): 60–66. https://doi.org/10.1016/j.nedt.2018.06.030.

Chartrand, G., M. Soucisse, P. Dubé, J. S. Trépanier, P. Drolet, and L. Sideris. "Self-Directed Learning by Video as a Means to Improve Technical Skills in Surgery Residents: A Randomized Controlled Trial." *BMC Medical Education* 21, no. 1 (2021): article 91. https://doi.org/10.1186/s12909-021-02524-y.

Garrison, D. Randy. "Self-Directed Learning: Toward a Comprehensive Model." *Adult Education Quarterly* 48, no. 1 (1997): 18–33.

Georgetown University School of Medicine. "Journeys Curriculum." Accessed January 28, 2022. https://som.georgetown.edu/curriculum/journeyscurriculum/.

Heck, Amber J., Courtney E. Cross, and Veronica Y. Tatum. "Early Medical Education Readiness Interventions: Enhancing Undergraduate Preparedness." In *Handbook of Research on the Efficacy of Training Programs and Systems in Medical Education*, edited by Ruth Gotian, Yoon Kang, and Joseph Safdieh, 283–304. Hershey, PA: IGI Global, 2020.

Hendricson, W. D., S. C. Andrieu, D. G. Chadwick, J. E. Chmar, J. R. Cole, M. C. George, G. N. Glickman, et al. "Educational Strategies Associated with Development of Problem-Solving, Critical Thinking, and Self-Directed Learning," *Journal of Dental Education* 70, no. 9 (2006): 925–36. https://doi.org/10.1002/j.0022-0337.2006.70.9.tb04163.x.

Hill, M., M. Peters, M. Salvaggio, J. Vinnedge, and A. Darden. "Implementation and Evaluation of a Self-Directed Learning Activity for First-Year Medical Students." *Medical Education Online* 25, no. 1 (2020): 1717780. https://doi.org/10.1080/10872981.2020.1717780.

International Society for Self-Directed Learning. "About Us." Accessed January 28, 2022. https://www.sdlglobal.com/about-us.

Jeong, D., J. Presseau, R. ElChamaa, D. N. Naumann, C. Mascaro, F. Luconi, K. M. Smith, and S. Kitto. "Barriers and Facilitators to Self-Directed Learning in Continuing Professional Development for Physicians in Canada: A Scoping Review." *Academic Medicine: Journal of the Association of American Medical Colleges* 93, no. 8 (2018): 1245–54. https://doi.org/10.1097/ACM.0000000000002237.

Knowles, Malcolm S. "Application in Continuing Education for the Health Professions: Chapter Five of 'Andragogy in Action.'" *Mobius* 5, no. 2 (1985): 80–100. https://doi.org/10.1002/chp.4760050212.

———. *Self-Directed Learning: A Guide for Learners and Teachers*. New York: Association Press, 1975.

Liaison Committee on Medical Education. *Functions and Structure of a Medical School: Standards for Accreditation of Medical Education Programs Leading to the MD Degree*. Washington, DC: Association of American Medical Colleges, 2021.

———. "Scope and Purpose of Accreditation." Accessed January 28, 2022. https://lcme.org/about/.

Lim, Y. S., V. T. Lyons, and J. M. Willey. "Supporting Self-Directed Learning: A National Needs Analysis," *Medical Science Educator* 31, no. 3 (2021): 1091–99. https://doi.org/10.1007/s40670-021-01278-y.

Murad, M. H., F. Coto-Yglesias, P. Varkey, L. J. Prokop, and A. L. Murad. "The Effectiveness of Self-Directed Learning in Health Professions Education: A Systematic Review." *Medical Education* 44, no. 11 (2010): 1057–68. https://doi.org/10.1111/j.1365-2923.2010.03750.x.

Ricotta, D. N., J. B. Richards, K. M. Atkins, M. M. Hayes, K. McOwen, M. I. Soffler, C. D. Tibbles, A. J. Whelan, R. M. Schwartzstein, and on behalf of Millennium Conference 2019 writing group. "Self-Directed Learning in Medical Education: Training for a Lifetime of Discovery." *Teaching and Learning in Medicine* (July 2021): 1–11. https://doi.org/10.1080/10401334.2021.1938074.

Simon, F. A., and C. A. Aschenbrener. "Undergraduate Medical Education Accreditation as a Driver of Lifelong Learning," *Journal of Continuing Education in the Health Professions* 25, no. 3 (2005): 157–61. https://doi.org/10.1002/chp.23.

Vector Solutions. "Teaching Attitudes: The Affective Domain of Learning and Learning Objectives." Accessed January 28, 2022. https://www.vectorsolutions.com/resources/blogs/teaching-attitudes-the-affective-domain-of-learning-and-learning-objectives/.

Wu, J. H., P. A. Gruppuso, and E. Y. Adashi. "The Self-Directed Medical Student Curriculum." *JAMA* 326, no. 20 (2021): 2005–6. https://doi.org/10.1001/jama.2021.16312.

Epilogue

EMPOWERING THE LIBRARY AS A PARTNER IN ACCREDITATION

Darell Schmick, Noorda College of Osteopathic Medicine

The previous pages of this book clearly demonstrate that libraries provide tremendous value to their institutions regarding the accreditation process. This value is enhanced by libraries reevaluating how they approach their institution's accreditation processes to be better partners. The library frequently is viewed as a natural collaborator within an organization and is involved with many different entities. As a result, the library can aid existing efforts in place for accrediting efforts and augment them in areas that may not have been previously identified.

Libraries benefit the accredited programs within their institutions by providing personnel, resources, and services that help with meeting accreditation standards. However, there are many areas an organization must address to demonstrate it is meeting accreditation standards. Within these standards, the library is not always explicitly mentioned. For example, many health sciences programs do not have specific library parameters that must be reported to their accrediting bodies. There are no requirements that dictate a minimum number of library staff, required services, or particular titles in the library's collection. The fact that the library is not mentioned does not mean the library is any less critical to the accreditation process. For those who do not have a fixed set of library-specific questions, the opportunities to demonstrate how the library fulfills other standards can be an elucidating experience for all and lead to new opportunities. Several chapters discuss this as a strategy. Further, what does a study of these standards signal for the library? Does this provide a chance to prioritize the library in ways not previously explored?

In reflecting on how your institution approaches accreditation and planning for the future, I recommend reflecting on previous iterations and writing down what you know. Reflecting on these past accreditation activities will require you to rely on your recollections and talk with other library staff who were involved. It would also be beneficial to gain further insight by speaking with stakeholders who have been involved with accreditation in the past. It will also be necessary, when possible, to read the report submitted for accreditation. During this time of reflection, try to answer the following questions:

- How did you feel about how the accreditation process was conducted?
- Do you believe the library had a proper voice in the process? If not, why?
- Are there opportunities for the library to be a better or more valuable partner in the accreditation process?
- Do you think the accreditation report provided a complete picture of the library's value to the organization? If not, what do you feel was left out?

And finally, write down what improvement(s) you wish for the next time around. Then, when reading (and rereading) these chapters for reference, make a note of where these teams were able to excel in areas that you wish to improve.

In addition to the narratives told by our chapter authors, be sure to review the supplemental content they provided. For example, some of our chapter authors have been gracious enough to share their survey and worksheet data in telling their accreditation stories. Utilize these or draw inspiration from them; they can be found in the appendix to follow.

As with any extensive, all-encompassing organizational effort, libraries have benefited from demonstrating their value to the stakeholders, patrons, and greater community.

Accreditation is a process that is no different. I challenge you to reflect on the stories shared within this book and how they apply to your institution.

Appendix

Following is the worksheet that students in the writing groups complete prior to meeting with the librarian, outlining a learning gap relating to their review topic; sources, search strategy, and citations relevant to the learning gap followed by the student assessment, outlining whether this process addressed the learning gap. The worksheet also includes the rubric from which the librarian assessed the responses from the individual students.

Name:

Embryology Paper Group Number:

Georgetown University School of Medicine Self-Directed Learning Student Worksheet[1] for Embryology Mini-review paper.

Purpose: This worksheet was designed to ensure that students meet the requirements for self-directed learning. This includes all of the following steps in order within a short time-frame[2]:

1) the medical student's self-assessment of his/her learning needs.
2) the medical student's independent identification, analysis, and synthesis of relevant information.
3) the medical student's appraisal of the credibility of information sources.
4) the facilitator's assessment of and feedback to the student on his/her information seeking skills.

Topic of your Mini-Review Paper:

Step 1: Identify your learning needs or a gap in knowledge you want to fill.

1. What do you want to learn that will help you to get information for your paper?

2. Where did you find the answer to your question?

Resource Searched: ☐ PubMed MEDLINE ☐ Ovid MEDLINE ☐ Textbook/eBook

☐ Other (specify)

3. List your Search Strategy. Which search terms did you use?

4. List 3 relevant citations gained from your search:

Citation #1:

Citation #2:

Citation #3:

1 Based on University of Illinois College of Medicine Self-Directed Learning Worksheet
2 LCME. Functions and Structure of a Medical School For Surveys in the 2021-2022 Academic Year. March 2020. Available from https://lcme.org/publications/, accessed 3/25/2022

1

Steps 2 and 3: Independent identification, analysis, and synthesis of relevant information; appraisal of the credibility of information sources

5. Analyze one of the three primary sources you listed above.

Citation #:

a. Strengths: What makes this information useful? What leads you to believe it?

b. Weaknesses: What are limitations of the information? What leads you to doubt it?

c. Did this source answer the learning gap listed in #1 above?

Upload the worksheet to Canvas HERE no later than [DUE DATE / TIME]

You will be evaluated based on the rubric on page 3. Feedback is formative only and does not count as part of your grade for the paper.

2

Step 4: Facilitator's assessment of and feedback to the student on his/her information seeking skills.

To be completed by the faculty evaluator

Criterion	Needs improvement	Meets expectations	Exceeds expectations
1. Identification of learning gap.	Learning gap not identified or unclear.	Learning gap identified but very general.	Learning gap specific and detailed.
2. Sources used to find information on paper topic.	Sources consulted were generalized resources, not focused on efficient access and retrieval of biomedical information, Retrieval includes anecdotal information, not peer-reviewed.	Some sources used included generalized search engines but did include sources providing retrieval from evidence-based, peer reviewed information.	All sources consulted to obtain information on paper topic provided access to high quality, evidence-based and peer-reviewed information.
3. Appropriate search strategy.	Search strategy did not contain relevant search terms and did not apply best practices for searching databases.	Search strategy contained some relevant search terms but also included terms which could result in retrieval not applicable to topic. Some best practices for searching databases were not used which would have resulted in more relevant retrieval.	Search strategy contained relevant search terms, clearly outlined with appropriate logic and is easily reproducible. Appropriate best practices for searching databases were used to generate a robust and relevant retrieval.
4. Analysis of selected source including strengths and weaknesses.	Sources are not evaluated. Strengths and weaknesses not described.	Strengths and weaknesses are described.	Strengths and weaknesses based on evidence-based medicine best practice methodology for evaluating an article.

Please provide short narrative feedback for each of the following questions.

1. Describe one thing the student/team did well regarding their information seeking and critical appraisal skills.

2. Describe one thing the student/team needs to improve upon regarding their information seeking and critical appraisal skills. Provide specific suggestion(s) for how to improve.

3

Index

Page references for figures are italicized.

ABOUT THE EDITOR

Darell Schmick, MLS, MBA, AHIP, has more than ten years of experience in academic medical libraries. He is currently the inaugural library director at Noorda College of Osteopathic Medicine; this is the second medical school in which he has played an involved role as director in establishing institutional accreditation. Mr. Schmick is an active member of the Medical Library Association and the Midcontinental Chapter of the Medical Library Association. As immediate past chair of the Osteopathic Caucus of the Medical Library Association, he has shepherded projects within the caucus to elevate the visibility of osteopathic librarians in schools of osteopathic medicine.

Previously, Mr. Schmick worked at the University of the Incarnate Word as founding director of the library for the School of Osteopathic Medicine, as research librarian at the University of Utah School of Medicine, and as information services librarian at the University of Missouri–Columbia School of Medicine. Mr. Schmick is a contributing author to previous Rowman & Littlefield publications such as *Transforming Health Sciences Library Spaces* and *Information and Innovation: A Natural Combination for the Health Sciences.*

ABOUT THE AUTHORS

Rhonda L. Altonen holds an MLS and MS in instructional design from Emporia State University and is the director of library services at the Touro College of Osteopathic Medicine and College of Pharmacy in Harlem. As the director of library services, she has been involved in the growth of the osteopathic medicine program at a new campus in Montana as well as a new Pathology Assistant (PathA) program opening on the Harlem campus. In addition, she and her staff have assisted in the transition of both teaching courses and providing student services in the virtual and hybrid formats during the COVID-19 closures. Prior to Touro, she worked as a reference and educational librarian at New York Medical College in Valhalla, New York, as the technical services librarian for the Culinary Institute in Hyde Park, New York, and was library director for the Unification Theological Seminary in New York City.

Charlotte M. Beyer, AHIP, is the associate vice president of the Boxer Library and Information Collaboration within the division of Academic and Faculty Affairs at Rosalind Franklin University of Medicine and Science (RFUMS) located in North Chicago, Illinois. In her position she facilitates the continuous transformation of the Boxer Library into an environment that promotes and supports the use of quality information as the foundation of the university's educational, research, and clinical activities and initiatives. She also shares her knowledge and expertise as part of the Academic and Faculty Affairs leadership team. Ms. Beyer received her master of science degree in information science from the State University of New York at Albany in 2007 before arriving at RFUMS as the instruction and reference librarian in 2010, a position she held until 2020. From 2020 to 2022, she held the title of library director. She has presented and published in areas such as information literacy, staff development, online learning, hybrid learning, universal design, accessibility, and evidence-based practice as well as being a distinguished member of the Academy of Health Information Professionals. In addition, she also holds faculty appointments within the College of Health Professions and the Chicago Medical School at RFUMS.

Jennifer Brown is the associate dean for academic affairs at Noorda College of Osteopathic Medicine. She came to the role after twenty years of work in exam preparation for standardized exams, specializing in physician and allied health licensure. She had the opportunity to work with dozens of institutions and thousands of students across the United States and the Caribbean to create study plans and academic support programs and to develop expertise in physician education programming and current challenges facing students, faculty, and administration at medical schools. Jennifer holds a master of science degree in higher education administration, a nutrition therapy practitioner degree, and a bachelor of the arts degree from Harvard College.

Roy Brown is a research and education librarian at the Health Sciences Library at Virginia Commonwealth University (VCU). He serves as liaison to VCU Health and the VCU School of Nursing nurses. As a liaison, he has participated in two Magnet reaccreditation processes and supports the evidence-based practice (EBP) and performance improvement initiatives nurses are doing in the clinical environment. He also works as an EBP immersion facilitator/librarian with the Helene Fuld Health Trust National Institute for Evidence-based Practice in Nursing and Healthcare at the Ohio State University School of Nursing. Roy has presented about his work with these groups, including successful EBP tools and strategies he utilizes, at the American Nurse Credentialing Center (ANCC) Magnet Conference, the ANCC Pathways to Excellence Conference, and other state and regional nursing conferences.

Susan B. Clark serves as director of the Rowland Medical Library and chair of Academic Information Services at the University of Mississippi Medical Center (UMMC). Ms. Clark works to develop the library as a place, as critical infrastructure, and as integrated partner with stakeholders at UMMC. She is particularly invested in positioning the library as an active partner in the educational, research, and clinical missions. She oversees the integration of information-seeking and lifelong learning skills into the curriculum of all seven schools housed at UMMC. Her previous roles at UMMC include head of reference and instruction. She received the master of librarianship degree from Emory University and holds memberships in various library associations statewide, regionally, and nationally.

Grant Connors is the associate director of education services for Dahlgren Memorial Library. One of the primary roles of his position is that of assistant course director for the Georgetown School of Medicine Evidence-Based Medicine course. Grant received his master's degree in library science from the University of North Texas and holds a certificate in copyright management from the Special Library Association. In addition, Grant teaches the Evidence-Based Medicine course for the Integrative Medicine and Health Sciences graduate program at Georgetown University Medical Center.

Ana Corral, MLIS, is a medical & health sciences librarian with the University of Houston's Health Sciences Library. She primarily supports the newly established College of Medicine with liaison services, research support, and evidence-based practices. Prior to the University of Houston, Ana was the community engagement & research librarian with the University Libraries at Virginia Tech, where she provided support for community-based research and initiatives. Ana is a former Medical Library Association Research Training Institute fellow and is in the process of completing her Level II Consumer Health Information Specialization from MLA/NLM. She earned a bachelor of arts degree in comparative literature and a bachelor of arts degree in interdisciplinary studies with a focus on gender in educational systems, both from the University of California-Berkeley, and a master of library and information science degree from Wayne State University. Her research interests include community-based participatory research methods and health information applications and the interaction between language, colonial research practices, and information access and dissemination.

Dr. John J. Dougherty is the founding dean and chief academic officer for the newly approved Noorda College of Osteopathic Medicine in Provo, Utah. Immediately before coming to Provo, Dr. Dougherty had been serving as dean of the medical school for Touro University in Henderson, Nevada. Prior to that he served in a variety of senior leadership roles at his alma matter in Kansas City for more than twenty years. Dr. Dougherty is a certified physician leader in administration. He completed a senior leadership development program and a national health policy fellowship, and holds a certificate in finance from the University of California-San Diego Rady School of Management.

Dr. G. Ian Gallicano is an associate professor in the department of Biochemistry and Molecular & Cellular Biology and the director of the Transgenic Core Facility at Georgetown University Medical Center in Washington,

DC. Dr. Gallicano has a PhD in zoology from Arizona State University and conducted a postdoctoral training fellowship at the University of Chicago, where he researched molecular biology including knockout and transgenic technologies. Dr. Gallicano is currently conducting research in the area of signaling in embryonic stem cells and the role of microRNAs.

Rachel Helbing, EdD, AHIP, is director of library services for the health sciences at the University of Houston. She has worked in consumer health, hospital, and academic health sciences libraries. Her interests include interprofessional education, clinical informatics, and evidence-based practice. Rachel earned a bachelor of arts degree in psychology from Miami University, as well as a master of library and information science and master of science in health informatics degrees, both from Kent State University. She was a member of the 2018–2019 cohort of the Medical Library Association's Rising Stars program and a member of the 2020–2021 cohort of the Cougar Chairs Leadership Academy. She completed an executive doctor of education degree in professional leadership with an emphasis in health science education from the University of Houston in 2022.

Yvonne M. Hernandez, PhD, is an associate professor of pharmacology and physiology and the associate dean for preclinical education at Georgetown University School of Medicine (GUSOM). For the past two decades, she has focused primarily on medical and graduate education, leading two iterations of reforms of the preclinical medical curriculum and developing novel preclinical courses and an innovative curriculum to introduce electronic health record and prescribing skills to preclinical students. She has been involved in three rounds of Liaison Committee on Medical Education (LCME) accreditation at GUSOM, holding leadership roles in the past two cycles.

Elizabeth G. Hinton is head of research impact and engagement and associate professor at the University of Mississippi Medical Center's Rowland Medical Library. She is library liaison to the School of Population Health and the School of Nursing, where she holds a secondary faculty appointment and is an accredited, trainer-certified reviewer for the Joanna Briggs Institute Comprehensive Systematic Review Training Program. Elizabeth is author or coauthor on multiple peer-reviewed journal articles, book and book chapters, posters, and papers, and is a peer reviewer for several journals. An active member in both the Medical Library Association and the Southern Chapter of the Medical Library Association, Elizabeth has held several leadership and committee appointments and is currently a senior member of the Academy of Health Information Professionals. Her professional interests include systematic reviews, library and educational assessment, and measuring publication output.

Sonya Lemke, MLS, AHIP, is the health sciences librarian at the Arkansas Colleges of Health Education, Taylor Health Sciences Library, in Fort Smith, Arkansas. She is the liaison to the College of Health Sciences, which currently consists of the physical therapy program, occupational therapy program, and the physician assistant program. She is the access services and systems librarian. She received her MLS from the University of North Texas, Denton, Texas. Upon graduating from library school in 2012, she worked for seven years in the biomedicine and pharmaceutical industry as an embedded librarian and then switched to academic librarianship in the summer of 2019. She serves in both the regional and national professional library organizations as an active member. She currently serves as secretary of the South-Central Chapter of the Medical Library Association Executive Board. Her professional interests are in health literacy, diversity and inclusion, and organizational behavior. Her personal interests are reading, photography, exercising, nature, and spending time with family and friends.

Connie Manning, MA, MLIS, AHIP, is a health sciences librarian at Taylor Health Sciences Library at Arkansas Colleges of Health Education and leads the management and assessment of electronic resources. She serves as the liaison librarian to the master of science in biomedicine and doctor of osteopathic medicine programs, as well as associated graduate medical education programs. Part of a team of three librarians at a new, stand-alone health education institution, she enjoys working at a small, growing library that provides exposure to all areas of library operations. Ms. Manning earned an MA in classics from Washington University in St. Louis and a MLIS with an archival studies concentration from the University of Wisconsin–Milwaukee. She has interned and worked in libraries, archives, and museums, including an archives internship with the American Center of Research in Amman, Jordan, in 2012 and an internship on copyright with Smithsonian Institution Libraries in 2015. She has received grant funding from organizations such as IMLS and NEH. She is an active member of regional and national medical library professional associations.

Dean Jett McCann has been the Dahlgren Memorial library director since 2007. His previous academic health sciences library positions include East Carolina University, Medical College of Georgia, and Medical University of South Carolina plus seven years' experience as an executive in the corporate world of library and publisher services. One of Dean McCann's charges when coming to Georgetown was to "weave the library into the curriculum," and the chapter he cowrote in this book is a perfect example.

Alison Montpetit is a PhD-prepared, registered nurse, distinguished fellow in the National Academies of Practice, and board certified in Nursing Professional Development. She serves as the current nursing director of clinical excellence at VCU Health and Magnet Program codirector, coleading VCU Medical Center in its fourth Magnet designation in 2020. She received her PhD and MS in adult nursing from the University of South Florida and BS in nursing from the University of North Carolina at Wilmington and completed a postdoctoral fellowship at VCU, bridging her basic science immunology training with her clinical practice background in intensive care nursing. Her program of research focused on exhaled breath biomarker characterization in mechanically ventilated, critically ill patients. In her current role, she leads an expert implementation team that supports organizational initiatives focused on nursing quality, research, evidence-based practice, performance improvement, innovation, professional practice, pain specialty, inpatient clinical research, and Magnet recognition.

Joanne M. Muellenbach is a health sciences library director with more than thirty years of hospital and academic health sciences library experience, including more than twenty years as a library administrator. Joanne is a graduate of the University of Wisconsin (UW), Madison, with a BA in English and an MA in library science. Over the course of her career, Joanne has served in a variety of health sciences library positions in Wisconsin; Colorado; Thunder Bay, Ontario, Canada; Pennsylvania; Nevada; and California, and she has had the unique opportunity to serve as the founding library director for four twenty-first-century medical schools. Currently, Joanne is the health sciences library director at California Health Sciences University, in Clovis, California.

Joanne grew up the second of six children in Milwaukee to a stay-at-home mom and a fashion designer dad who specialized in weddings and formal wear. As a result, she learned the valuable skill of sewing beginning at age eight. This inspired Joanne to pursue studies in apparel design and theatre, until she discovered that the only paid staff in the Milwaukee Repertory Theatre's costume shop where she volunteered was the lead designer! As a UW undergrad, a weekend trip to attend her cousin's women's ice hockey tournament in Minnesota changed her life. Joanne's passion for playing women's ice hockey spanned more than twenty years and took her to skating rinks in Wisconsin; Illinois; Minnesota; Colorado; and Ontario, Canada. Other interests include quilt making, bicycling, and staying in touch with family and friends throughout the United States and Canada.

Mitzi R. Norris serves as the executive director for academic effectiveness at the University of Mississippi Medical Center (UMMC). She oversees UMMC's academic accreditation activities for the Southern Association for Colleges and Schools Commission on Colleges as the liaison and for fourteen discipline-specific accreditations. She also leads the development of new academic programs, assessment, and continuing education. Dr. Norris has taught at institutions of higher learning for more than twenty-three years and has been involved with clinical education and continuing education for more than twenty-eight years. She is professor of health administration and teaches leadership. Previously she served as the educational director for a regional network of ten medical centers, encompassing eight states and 17,000 employees. She received her BS and MS in microbiology from Mississippi University for Women. Her PhD, from the University of Mississippi, is in educational leadership.

Douglas L. Varner (https://orcid.org/0000-0002-1963-8798) is the assistant dean for information management at Dahlgren Memorial Library, the Graduate Health & Life Sciences research library at Georgetown University Medical Center. His research interests include quantitative and qualitative assessment of the library value to institutional research and educational initiatives and the development of continuous quality improvement methodology to evaluate information services.

Dr. Jeff Weinfeld is a professor in the Georgetown University Department of Family Medicine. In the department he serves as director of medical student education and runs the evidence-based medicine course and DC Health Equity Longitudinal Integrated Clerkship. He has held positions in quality and informatics for governmental, nonprofit, and community organizations, including working with HRSA's Office of Health Information Technology and MedStar's Health Quality Office. He is board certified in family medicine and clinical informatics and practices at MedStar Family Medicine at Spring Valley in northwest Washington, DC. He received his medical degree from Boston University School of Medicine, completed his Family Medicine residency at the Georgetown University/Providence Hospital program, and received a master's degree in biomedical informatics from the Oregon Health & Science University. His interests include evidence-based medicine, medical education, caring for underserved patients, clinical decision support, and clinical informatics.

Michele L. Whitehead, MLS, MA, CSML, joined the Gibson D. Lewis Health Science Library at the University of North Texas (UNT) Health Science Center at Fort Worth (HSC) in early 2011, where she is currently the associate director of research, education, and engagement. Michele also serves as a faculty member at Tarleton State University in the Department of Criminology, Criminal Justice, and Public Administration.

Michele previously served as a faculty member at the University of Texas at Arlington (UTA) and began her education career in K–12 with Lubbock ISD. She holds two master's degrees: the first in criminology and criminal justice from UTA and the second in library science from UNT. She was also a member of the first cohort to complete the graduate certificate in school management and leadership at Harvard.

www.ingramcontent.com/pod-product-compliance
Ingram Content Group UK Ltd.
Pitfield, Milton Keynes, MK11 3LW, UK
UKHW041103150926
475561UK00001BA/12

9 781538 165577